Beautiful
ENCORE

Beautiful
ENCORE

MAKEOVERS *for* MATURE WOMEN

ANNE REIZER

Featuring Original Photography by
GABRIELA LAVALLE

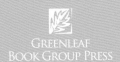

GREENLEAF
BOOK GROUP PRESS

Published by Greenleaf Book Group Press
Austin, Texas
www.gbgpress.com

Distributed by Greenleaf Book Group

For ordering information or special discounts for bulk purchases, please contact Greenleaf Book Group at PO Box 91869, Austin, TX 78709, 512.891.6100.

Design and composition by Greenleaf Book Group
Cover design by Greenleaf Book Group
Cover photography by Gabriela Lavalle
Interior photography by Gabriela Lavalle

Publisher's Cataloging-In-Publication Data
Reizer, Anne, 1944-
   Beautiful encore : makeovers for mature women / Anne Reizer ; featuring original photography by Gabriela Lavalle.—First edition.
     pages : illustrations ; cm
   Issued also as an ebook.
   ISBN: 978-1-62634-135-7
   1. Beauty, Personal. 2. Older women—Health and hygiene. I. Lavalle, Gabriela. II. Title.
RA778 .R45 2015
646.7/042   2014939457

Part of the Tree Neutral® program, which offsets the number of trees consumed in the production and printing of this book by taking proactive steps, such as planting trees in direct proportion to the number of trees used: www.treeneutral.com

TreeNeutral®

Printed in China on acid-free paper

14 15 16 17 18 19   10 9 8 7 6 5 4 3 2 1

First Edition

To Mike, for his unwavering support.

Contents

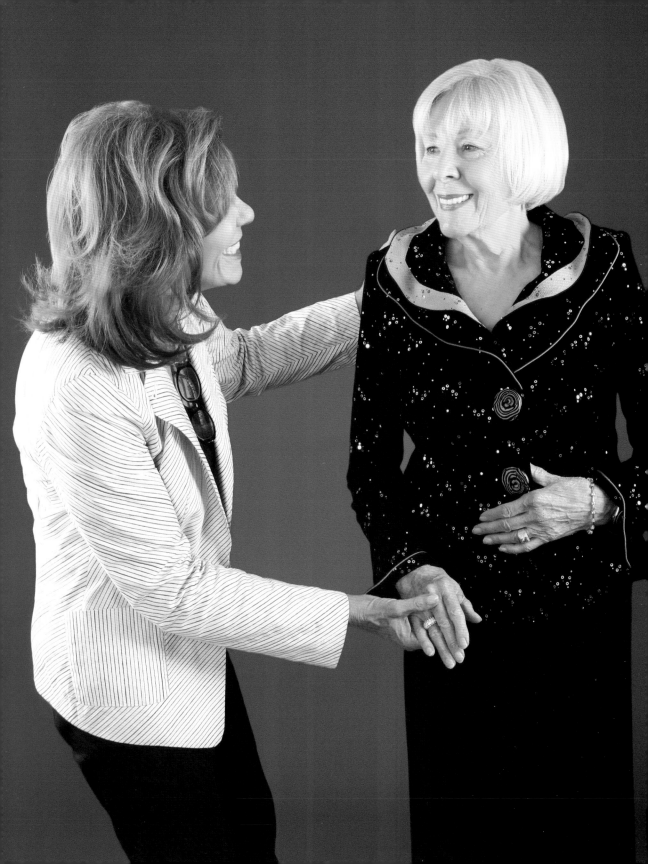

Introduction

" ... if you want to talk about where beauty really comes from, let's talk about brains and discipline. Because a woman with these qualities can do a lot toward making herself very, very attractive."

—*Aileen Mehle, also known as Suzy Knickerbocker*

You look sensational! Not often enough are mature women the recipients of this compliment. *Beautiful Encore* shows you that looking sensational is not as difficult as you might think, and that in making yourself look sensational, you will be presenting your **best** and **most authentic** self, the person you truly are.

It's time to reconsider your visual presentation, which will give you more confidence to meet new experiences gracefully.

Not one of us has "come of age" without weathering bumpy periods and having to make adjustments to a life's plan. Each of us has matured through the life events that have shaped our characters. Now, as we meet new and inevitable challenges and opportunities, we can draw on a lifetime of experiences.

It's time to reconsider your visual presentation, which will give you more confidence to **MEET NEW EXPERIENCES GRACEFULLY.**

Women in our generation have worn all manner of clothing and hairstyles in our lifetimes. We spent our twenties in miniskirts. We have worn culottes, maxi dresses, wrap dresses, dresses that looked like nightgowns, power suits with dramatic shoulder pads, western and bohemian styles. We have idolized women like Jacqueline Kennedy Onassis and Audrey Hepburn. Why are we now limiting our style and grooming to a much more narrow menu? Do we feel minimized by our ages? Do we feel that only young women have a right to feel beautiful? Have we decided, for the sake of convenience, to give up—to let apathy dictate that we let go of our curiosity and our commitment to looking good?

When appearance becomes an afterthought, it quickly leads to no thought. Without a polished exterior, your interior is in shadow. Illuminating yourself by caring about your hair, clothing, makeup, and most important of all your health is neither a superficial pursuit nor an insurmountable goal. You can project a visual language that says to your peers that you're comfortable and confident in who you've become. **Looking good is not a superficial endeavor! It leads to engagement and success in other facets of your life.** Keeping yourself current and put-together in your mature years tells those who interact with you that you're engaged and have a plan for your time. **Investing in ourselves helps us project confidence and reinforces how we want to be perceived.**

Being meticulous with skin care and makeup application and experimenting with new clothing and hairstyles might seem to require too much effort. But let me tell you, it's worth it! We are bombarded in the marketplace by the assertion that we should fight the signs of aging. Still, we know that we can't halt it altogether. **So let's embrace our maturity, harness our life experiences, and acquire the right tools and techniques for taking care of ourselves.** Products we used at forty may not be appropriate for our delicate skin. Perhaps you are considering a new hairstyle—maybe coloring your hair or embracing your gray. Or maybe you're not sure if you can wear a patterned dress or trendy jeans? Inevitably, you have new health concerns that are likely related to age, rather than to disease. Use these questions to ignite the spark of curiosity that will lead you to reach out to experts who can guide us toward presenting our best selves.

I am thrilled to be my age and I want every one of you to be, too. Let *Beautiful Encore* inspire you to discover your mature style.

———

Beautiful Encore is not a how-to book. It's a catalyst to empower you to reinvest in yourself, physically and emotionally. It presents inspiration for exploring hair, makeup, and apparel choices.

We've chosen real women to be our models—each with a different story, body type, and lifestyle. Each woman has the ingredients so necessary for change: curiosity and a positive attitude. This view of life is one that has not always come easily. In many cases these models have found the inner strength to weather challenges and, in the process, transform themselves and flourish.

What they all have in common is that each of them came to the Beautiful Encore project open to the belief that a polished presentation was worth the risk of allowing stylists to take full control. The results speak for themselves. For me, as the project facilitator, the "oh my" moment was overwhelming, when each woman saw her newly styled look.

Professional stylists and makeup artists have helped the models discover which makeup palette and haircut best suit their faces and hair textures. Stylists have helped choose clothing that fits and flatters their body types. It's important to note that it's not the price tag on the garment that has changed a model's appearance; it's the effect of the thoughtful, individual choices made in assembling her look.

I want every woman in my generation to enjoy the visibility and confidence of an individual style. Once we learn that our visual appearance leads to increased self-assurance, we can harness the energy to pursue our new personal and professional goals.

—**Anne Reizer**

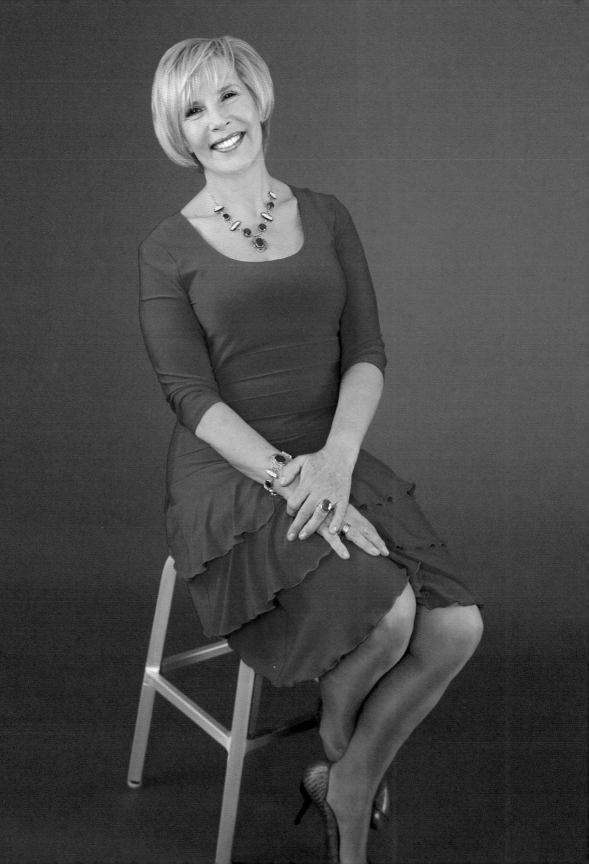

NATALIA

LOVER OF EDUCATION AND CULTURE

Age: 63   Height: 5' 3"

Natalia feels lucky to have been born in the remarkable Russian city of Saint Petersburg. She graduated from one of the city's oldest and most prestigious schools, the Second Saint Petersburg Gymnasium. Her love of travel, history, art, music, and languages sprang from her years as a student. As a girl, Natalia especially admired Nikolai Miklouho-Maclay's drawings depicting blue oceans and green palms, which she viewed during her many visits to the State Hermitage Museum. This artwork inspired her to become a traveler herself and escape the cold Russian winters.

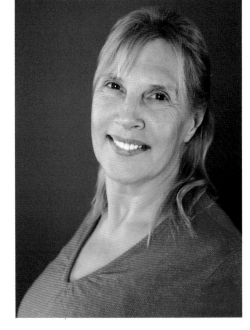

In the nineties, her husband's job was transferred and the family moved to Mexico City. Natalia attended the Universidad Nacional Autónoma de México to study Spanish, in order to better communicate in her new community. She was thrilled to be exposed to a completely different culture and environment. She found that by having a good attitude, staying busy with work, and being open to the unfamiliar, a family can thrive in a new

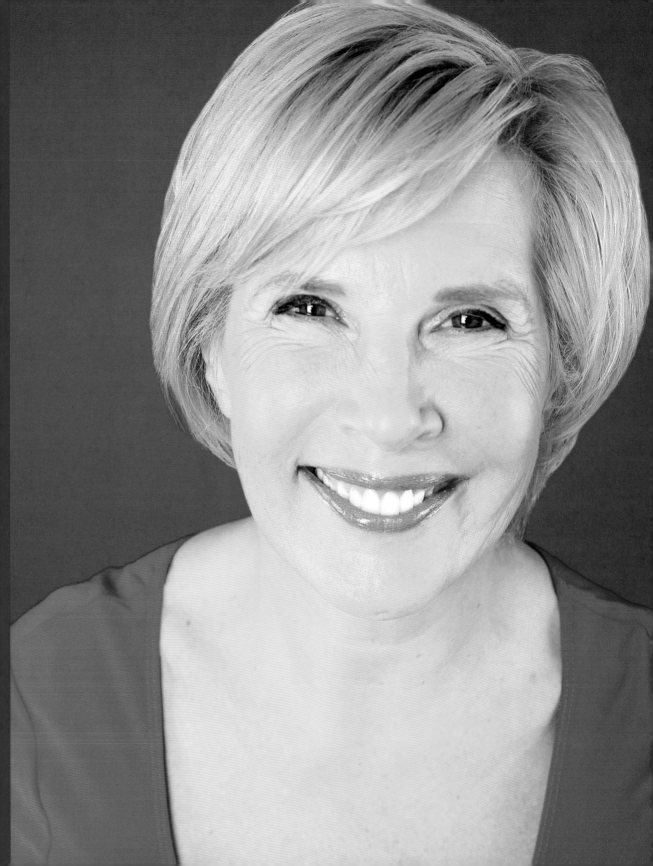

life in a different country. She now lives in Texas and teaches English as a second language at the college level. She adores her work; in the classroom she encounters students from many cultures from whom she learns something new each day.

Natalia and her husband miss cross-country skiing in the Russian snow, but they have taken up swimming instead, as it is better suited to Texas weather. She travels to Russia every summer to visit one of her two daughters, her grandchildren, and her sisters.

"I think that in order to **AGE GRACEFULLY** it is important to acknowledge the changes that occur in your body and mind and accept and embrace them."

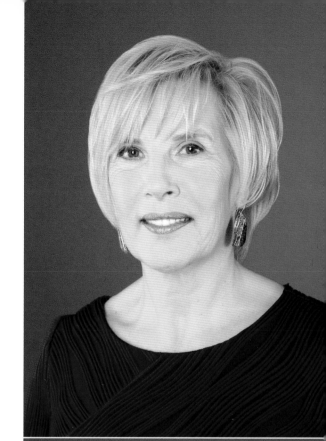

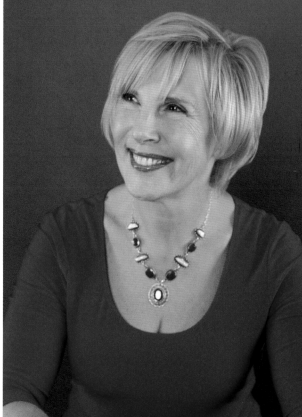

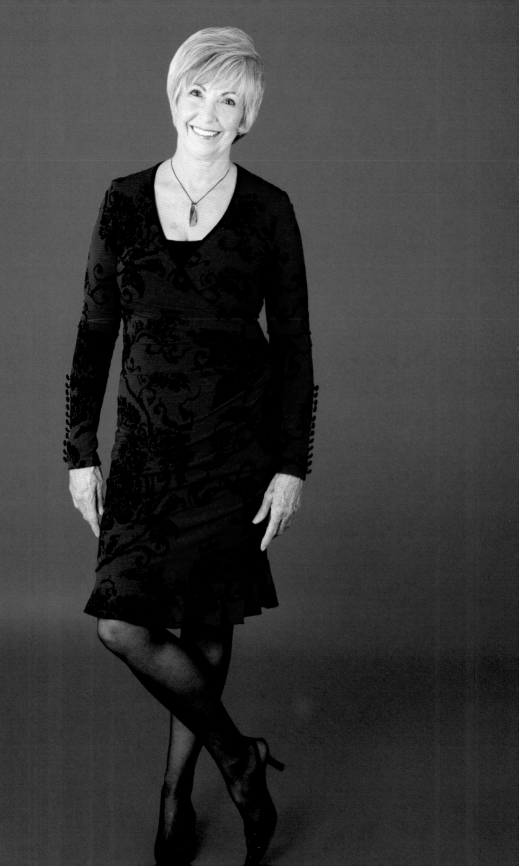

CHERYL

MASTER GARDENER AND COMMUNITY SUPPORTER

Age: 67   Height: 5' 4"

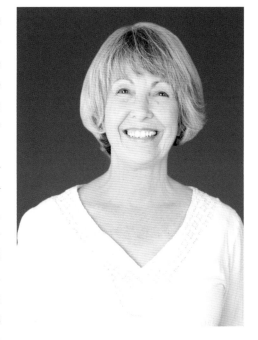

Cheryl has lived her entire life in the same part of Texas. There she met her husband of over forty years and raised three daughters, who all continue to reside in the area. In fact, she and her husband still live in the same home that their daughters grew up in.

Cheryl has been a small business owner for the past thirty-five years. After her father's tragic death in an auto accident, there were no sons to take over the family towing business. Cheryl stepped up and took over, running it for the next ten years. She knew she loved working directly with people, so after considering many options she then decided to go into the insurance business. Her honesty and genuine concern for others made her agency successful. After more than twenty years in the insurance industry, she retired.

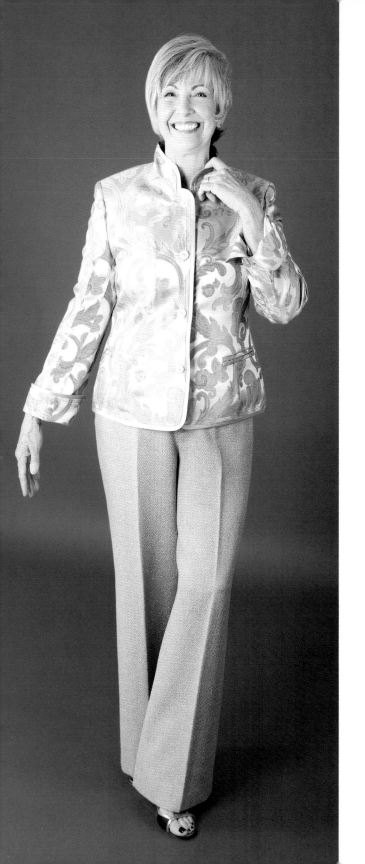

Despite her retirement, Cheryl can't quite slow down. She earned the highly esteemed designation of Master Gardener, which calls for a great deal of studying, course work, and volunteering. Being a Master Gardener provides her with the opportunity to give back to her community by supplying support and information about gardening.

Cheryl and her husband stay active in their church and enjoy traveling, especially to their vacation home on the beach in Galveston, where her entire family loves to get together. She feels blessed to be so involved in the lives of her eight grandchildren.

"STAYING BUSY IS JUST A WAY OF LIFE for both of us, sometimes as a couple, other times with our separate interests."

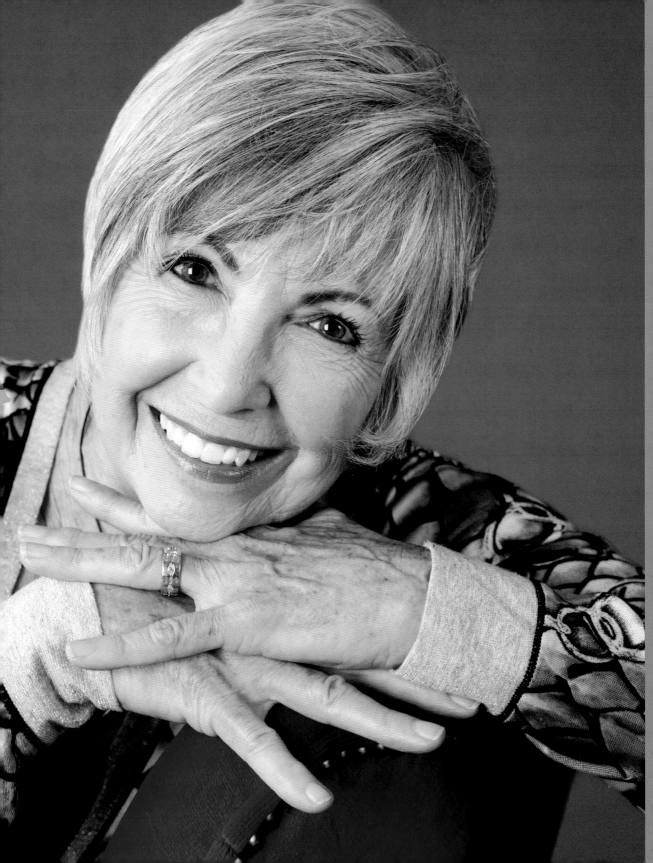

Older Wiser Happier

PAMELA BENISON, MA

My journey has been shaped by my efforts to follow the joy of discovery and accomplishment. Now, at age sixty-four, I realize that my enlightenment has come from persistence in rising to challenges. Hardships have been a part of my life. But resourcefulness when confronting heartache, loss, pain, and illness has helped me face adversities and my aging process. When I'm rising to meet a challenge, my inner strength guides me. In my quest to see the truth of a situation, I accept all of my feelings, not just the pleasurable ones. I treat myself with compassion and tenderness, making time and space to work things out rather than expecting myself to heal immediately. I feel resilient, because I welcome challenges as opportunities to grow and be happier.

Since the start of my psychotherapy practice, I have guided clients through challenges of their own: depression, anxiety, emotional and physical abuse, addictions, developmental passages, and relationship issues. In 1993 I formed Integrated Wellness, Inc. (www.pamela benison.com), as a teaching agency to help people face challenges by bringing forth the knowledge that arises from meditation, Gestalt therapy, cognitive behavioral therapy, positive psychology, and breathing and centering techniques that are rooted in the connection of mind and body. The key to adult happiness lies in connecting with others in meaningful ways, and that starts with building an effective sense of self.

How do we handle the challenges that are a part of life? How can we gain the confidence to move past them, accept ourselves as we are, and achieve true wellness? The "Challenges and Skills" graph represents a guide for seeing yourself during times of challenge and accessing positive skills you may already possess and turn a challenge into a confidence builder.

As challenges present themselves, our fluctuating skills move us along a continuum of resiliency and stress, depending on our level of confidence. That confidence is built on inner resourcefulness—the attitude that defines how we optimally face a challenge.

Challenge + Resourcefulness = Resilience

Or we see the opposite:

Challenge + Lack of Resourcefulness = Stress

The key is seeking and truly utilizing your own wise counsel. The old adage applies: Be true to yourself.

The Challenges

Let's take a look at the challenges women face at all stages of life.

DISCONNECTION FROM SELF AND OTHERS

One challenge women tend to face is not really knowing what makes them tick.

Life becomes meaningless when you don't know what makes *you* happy and fulfilled. Symptoms of malaise may include watching too much TV, isolating oneself and disinterest in socializing or communicating with loved ones, or giving in to negative self-talk. A woman stuck in this state of mind is unable to recognize

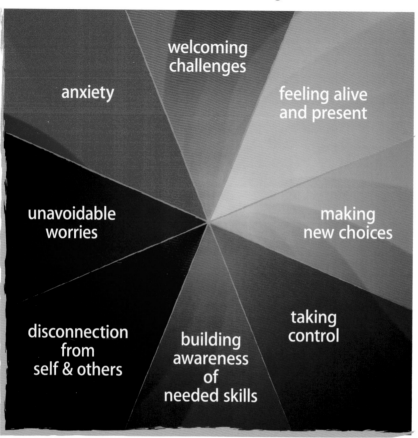

challenge + resource=resilience

welcoming challenges

anxiety

feeling alive and present

challenges

unavoidable worries

making new choices

disconnection from self & others

building awareness of needed skills

taking control

challenge + no resources=stress

skills

Designed by Dashiell Benison. "Challenges and Skills" graph from a lecture at the Integrative Medicine Conference, July 2013, presented by Mihaly Csikszentmihalyi. All the inner material has been adapted by Pamela Benison.

her resources nor access her deep well of resourcefulness.

The woman who finds herself in this vulnerable state must remember that making just **one simple change** can lead to a pathway out of lethargy.

UNAVOIDABLE WORRIES

Perhaps even more predictable among women are those inevitable day-to-day worries and anxiety. What are the unavoidable worries of life? We may worry about our finances, our health, our adult children and their problems, or just aging in general. When we worry too much, it can take over our whole life, leading to anxiety, which is a consistently worried state of mind. Anxiety is a clue that indicates new movement is needed. There have been studies on stress that reveal that *how* we think about stress matters. If your heart is pounding, teach yourself to say, "This is my body helping me rise to this challenge." Your body will believe you. Researchers found that the participants who said this to themselves had blood vessels that were relaxed and not constricted, and their hearts' vascular systems looked like they would in moments of joy and courage.

The Skills

The following skills help us build resources and avoid stress as we move through the challenges of aging.

BUILDING AWARENESS

As we age, we may say things like "I look old and ugly" or "I don't have a purpose"— we impose a negative story on ourselves. Yet what better time to create a new, positive story about your next stage in life? When you get stuck in old stories or roles, your energy is greatly diminished. Instead, ask yourself, "How do I want to live this moment?" and "What happens when there is no one else to please but me?" Address any thoughts that have made you anxious about your body or your purpose. Ask "How do I want to feel?" and "Why do I feel this way?" **The time for a change is now.**

TAKING CONTROL

How do we support ourselves more consciously? One way is by soothing yourself with answers from your deepest wisdom. Access the soothing energy within you by touching one of the three centers of the body: belly, diaphragm (area below the breasts), or heart. Each will have a distinctive message for you. Do the following exercise on a regular basis, and you will find that you have developed into your own personal psychologist.

Place your palms on your belly, the center of feminine power. Think of an issue that undermines your power. Breathe deeply and feel the space in your belly as you inhale and exhale. Then, with each exhale, empty yourself of stress. Delight in connecting with your breath. Imagine you are your own best friend. Say to yourself, "What is the most important energy I need to empower me?" Welcome the response and be patient—an answer will come to you.

Close your eyes, breathe, and touch your diaphragm. Become aware of the fear that haunts you. Ask yourself, "What do I need to support myself?" **When you** are fearful, the diaphragm feels knotted and tight.** When the diaphragm is relaxed, however, it is a source of profound support. Breathe slowly and deliberately, and let an answer emanate from this physical site into your consciousness. Accept the message of support. Feel the confidence that comes when you are vulnerable and honest.

Finally, touch your chest and breathe. Humbly acknowledge your love essence. Explore what your heart is telling you. Ask your heart, "How can I embrace what is loving for me?" Remember, your heart's job is to care for all your joys and sorrows. So learn to trust its wisdom, and remember that you are not alone. The heart combines strength, joy, and love, holding us together when we are grieving a loss or heartbreak that seems unending. The heart teaches us to open up to love again and again. But first you must open up to your heart.

Each of your three centers—belly, diaphragm, heart—is a site of strength. As we learn to use and trust these centers, we develop resiliency. **Practice turning inward for answers daily.**

MAKING NEW CHOICES

How do we know when we've acquired the skill of making bold, new choices? Let your emotions be your feedback system:

When you make a choice that rewards you with warm regard for yourself, it will promote confidence and well being. If you feel badly about a choice you've made, it was probably based on poor self-judgment, criticism, or feelings of unreasonable obligation.

Sometimes we need to change external conditions before we can see internal change.

Feeling purposeful is basic to making new choices. Start by looking for the inner values that have guided your life—the subtle manifestations that have determined your choices thus far. Have you taken good care of your health? Nurtured your relationships? Mastered your particular talents? Tended your spirituality? **Reflect on your life, and welcome a sense of awe at what you have accomplished.** Then continue to make choices that embody your inner values. Remember, confidence is built with an "I can" attitude. **As you make new choices, take charge of the variables within your control and let go what of you cannot control.**

Each of us has particular talents, strengths, and potential. When we feel resilient and resourceful, we are self-assured, imbued with value that reflects who we are. Our actions and words leave a positive imprint on others. This deep regard for ourselves and others shines brightly. We emit an intrinsic presence that is unique and actualized, even palpable. In this state, we feel a connection to our true self and to others. We are grateful for all we experience and all we are given. When we are **alive** in this way, we forget everything but the present moment. Whether we are dancing, bowling, reading, playing music, teaching, or having great sex, we are doing what we love and feeling vibrant.

WELCOMING CHALLENGES

The final skill to work on is a difficult one: actually welcoming the challenges of aging. We can build upon the skill of feeling alive and present as it allows us to see challenges as opportunities to grow. When we welcome challenges, we use less negative self-talk. As the philosopher Nietzsche explains, there is a "love of one's fate"—an acceptance of life's deepest sorrows, including chronic illness and death. As we grieve, we learn to feel grateful that we have had many wonderful moments with a friend, a spouse, a child. There is a joy in knowing we have shared life deeply with another.

As you look back on the challenges of your life so far, how have they expanded your confidence, your understanding, and your loving connections? How did they change your life in a positive way? Eleanor Roosevelt said, "You gain strength, courage, and confidence by every experience in which you really stop to look fear in the face. You are able to say to yourself, 'I lived through this horror. I can take the next thing that comes along.'"

So, my advice to you is to do the thing you think you cannot do. Discover the resources within. Get involved in life. Take control of your situation. Make new choices. Feel alive each moment. Welcome all challenges. As Peter Ustinov said, "The whole idea of living is to believe the best is yet to be." By developing the skills I have described here, you will find that you can rise to meet these challenges and create a happy, healthy future.

Say to yourself,
"WHAT IS THE MOST IMPORTANT ENERGY I NEED TO EMPOWER ME?"

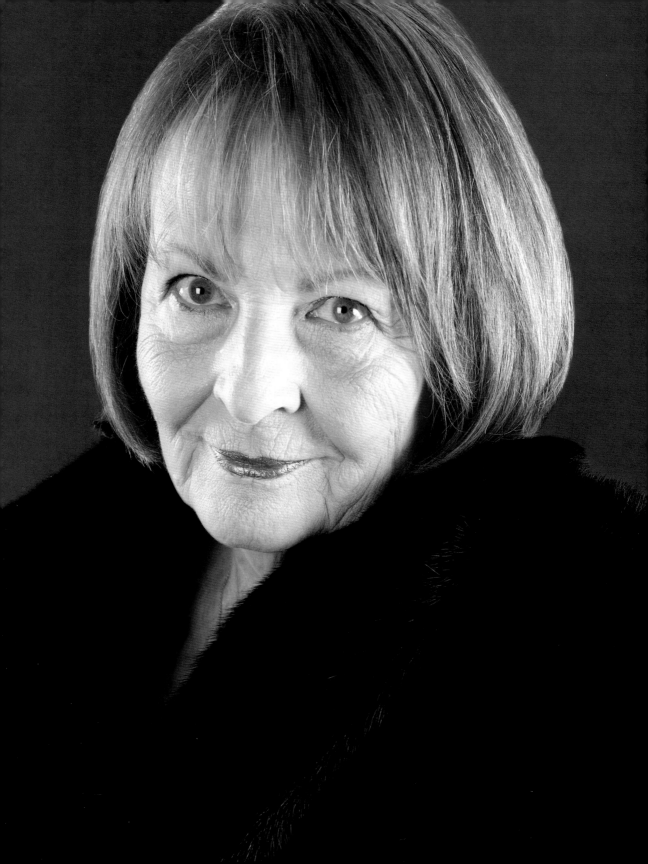

ELIZABETH

MASTER SEAMSTRESS AND TRUE TEXAN

Age: 75   Height: 5' 4"

Elizabeth was born an only child in Fort Worth and raised in Arlington, Texas. In fact, her mother's grandfather is the man who wrote to Congress to suggest that the city be named Arlington. She's a Texan through and through. Elizabeth met and married her husband while at the University of Texas, and the two had four children.

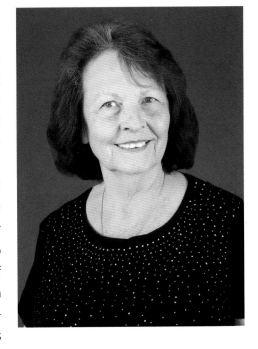

Elizabeth loves sewing. She held several positions in the fashion industry, including wholesale selling to the trade. With her knowledge of sewing, she developed a deep understanding of the fit and construction of garments. Her expertise led her to design and sew her daughters' and daughter-in-law's wedding dresses. After her husband's death in 2009, Elizabeth was asked to work as a seamstress at her friend's custom drapery and home accessories company. At seventy-five, Elizabeth continues to work with her hands, maintaining her position as a master seamstress. She also has a real estate license and completes several transactions a year, but her true love is sewing. Age

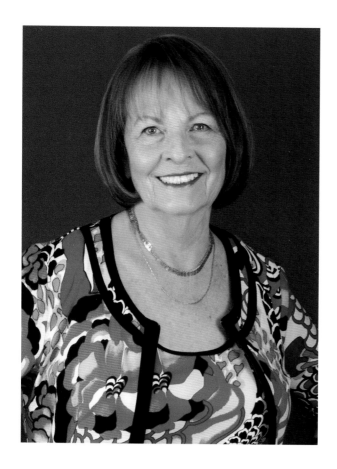

is no barrier to her creativity or success.

Elizabeth cherishes her involvement in her beloved national fraternity, Zeta Tau Alpha, and she has been an alumna adviser at Arlington State College, the University of Kentucky, and Southern Methodist University. She was also asked by the national council to become the national standards adviser for Zeta and has served as the convention chairman at the national convention.

Elizabeth attributes her longevity, good fortune, and happiness to her faith in God.

"I feel that age is a frame of mind and truly believe that **YOU ARE ONLY AS OLD AS YOU LET YOURSELF FEEL.**"

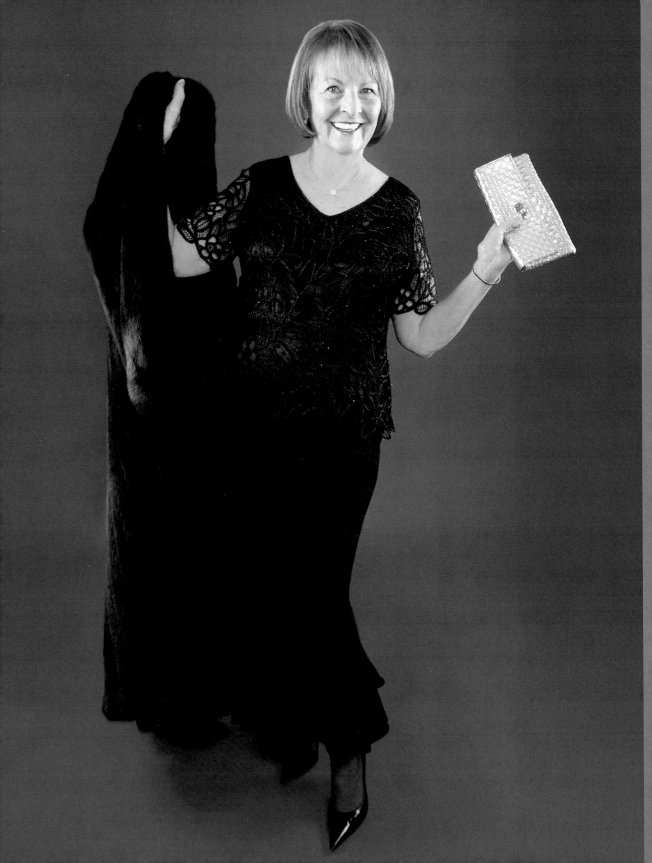

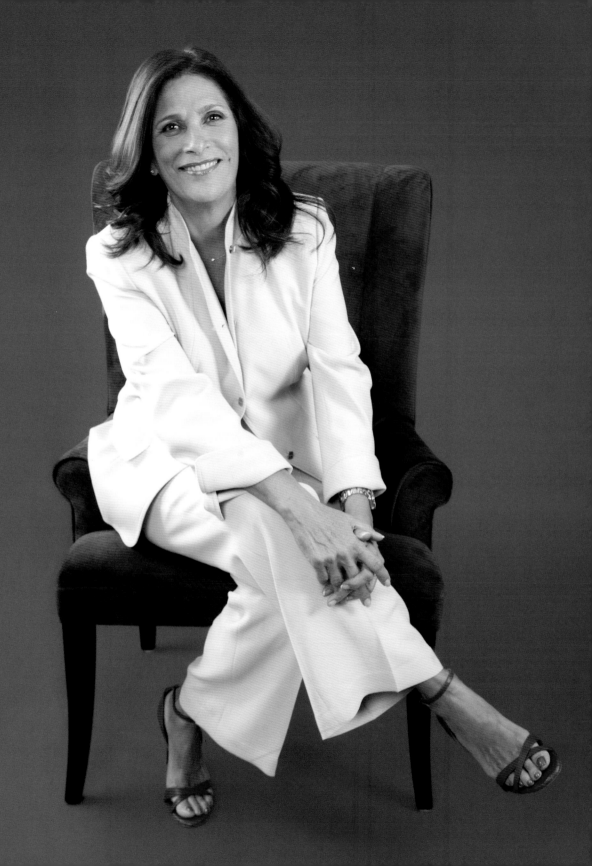

CHAGUA

LOVING MOTHER AND EDUCATOR

Age: 62   Height: 5' 7"

Chagua began working as a Montessori teacher after she was married. Together with her sister, she owned and managed a Montessori school in Mexico for eleven years. When her fourth child was born with special needs—later diagnosed as PDD-NOS, autism spectrum—she accepted and faced the challenge with love, despite the difficult and exhausting routines. She and her family moved from Mexico to the United States to seek better opportunities for her youngest son. She is now grandmother to seven grandchildren. She feels blessed and grateful to have watched her family grow.

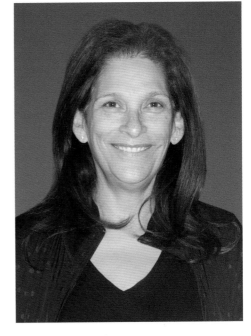

Chagua is honest when she evaluates her life and its priorities, accepting the need to rebalance when she sees an aspect that can be improved. Knitting is Chagua's passion, and she pours her creativity and vision into each piece she makes. She also practices meditation, which gives her a calm perspective on life. She believes that living in the present is the key to happiness and joy. Through her quiet pursuits Chagua has lived each day to the fullest.

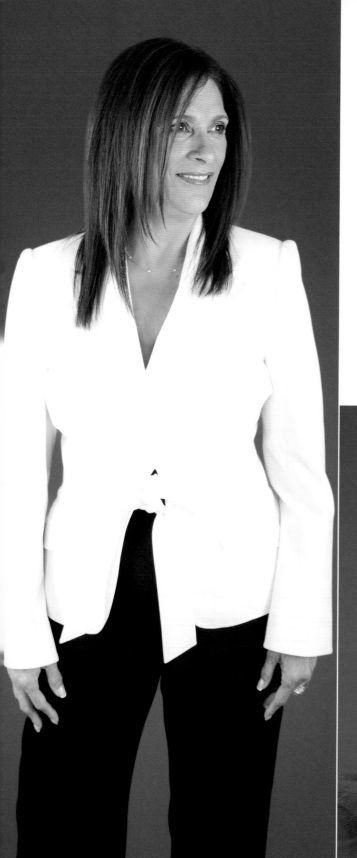

"I have realized that the most precious moments come only from **LIVING IN THE PRESENT,** not regretting the past, nor having false expectations for the future."

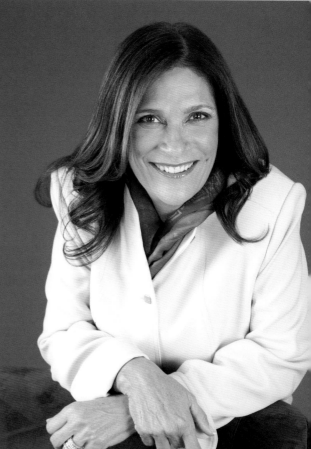

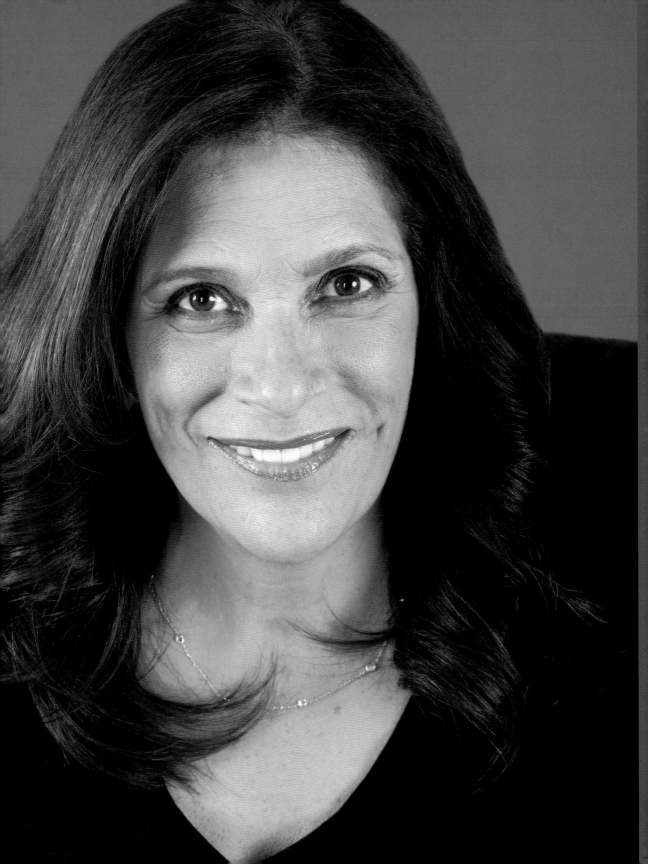

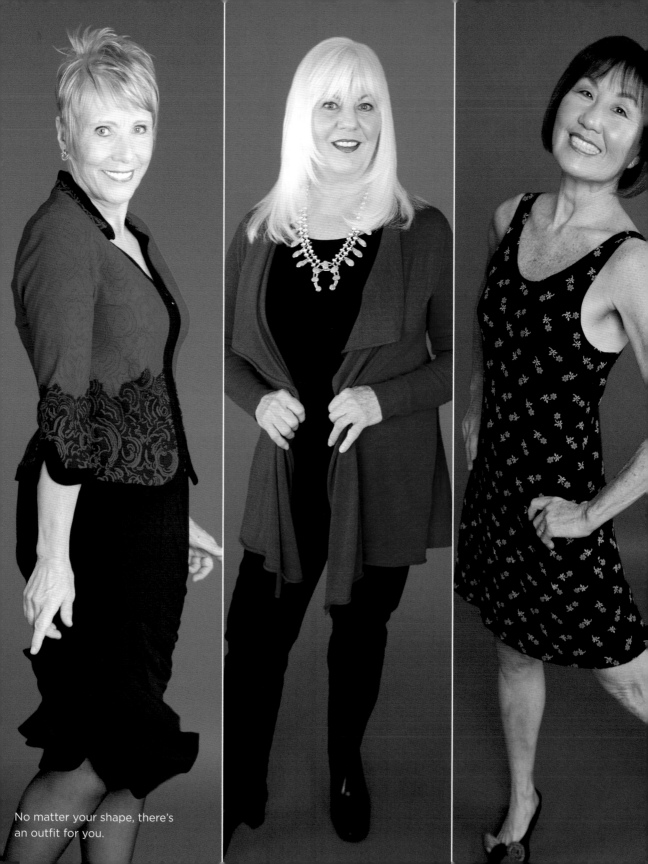

No matter your shape, there's an outfit for you.

Refresh Your Wardrobe

LINDA DIETERT, WARDROBE STYLIST

As a boutique owner, I have the job of dressing women of all ages in clothes that make them feel beautiful, comfortable, and that are lifestyle appropriate. One suggestion I have for mature women is to draw style inspiration from women their own age, like Meryl Streep, Dame Judy Dench, Diane Keaton, and Oprah Winfrey. All are beautiful and stylish and always look put together. Or perhaps you have a stylish friend. Use her look as inspiration! She will be flattered.

Take a close look at your wardrobe. Purge your closet of items that have stains, have fabric pills, or no longer fit you. Making sure your garments

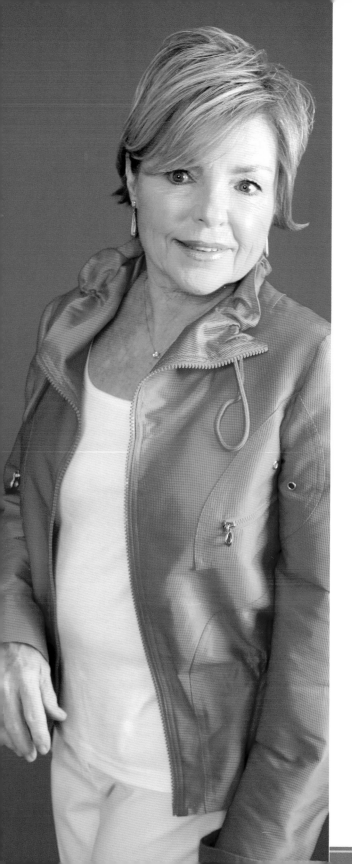

don't appear worn out or dated is of utmost importance in presenting a polished look.

Vintage is a big trend these days, and as tempting as it may be to pull out and wear those items from decades past, we must be careful not to miss the mark and simply look outdated. My advice is to avoid wearing the original piece—most likely, the fit and cut will be off. It is important to stay current with your choices. If you have a piece that you simply can't part with, consider having it updated by a tailor.

As far as following the trends, I encourage you to go for it, as long as you feel confident and comfortable. Never feel like trends are inaccessible to you because of your age. If you feel good in a pair of skinny jeans, wear them! As long as you feel good about yourself in whatever you're wearing, the sky is the limit.

Playing with a new color in your wardrobe is a good way to update or refresh your look. Don't be afraid of black—it's classic and looks great on everybody. The perfect little black dress with just the right accessories is a tried-and-true look, perfect for any occasion. I also encourage you to experiment with color. If you love red, wear it. If you love purple, wear it. Royal blue is a great color—it stands out, and it's happy. If you are unsure about wearing bolder colors in a pant or a top, try accessorizing with them in scarves, shoes, or purses. A pop of color will really complete your look. Using color is how you can really let your personality shine in fashion.

As long as you feel good about yourself in whatever you're wearing, **THE SKY IS THE LIMIT.**

Many women think they have to break the bank to dress well, but that's just not true. There is no need to spend a lot of money to look great. Some of the best-dressed women are bargain shoppers. The hunt is part of the fun, and it pays off! Remember, always look closely at the quality of the fabric, the print, and the cut of your garments.

I admit, some of my own favorite pieces were a bit costly, but I have worn them time and time again. They were true investments! I recommend investing in a few classic staple pieces for your own wardrobe. A good pair of black pants is essential. Look for quality fabric and a flattering fit. If you have to pay a little bit more for the perfect pair of black pants, it will be worth it in the long run. Also, invest in a good pair of jeans. An unflattering pair of jeans will make you look out of date. Look for something in a current color wash that's comfortable and looks good on you. If you're unsure, take a friend and ask her opinion. Or consult with the boutique staff—their job is to make you look and feel great!

I challenge you to step out of your comfort zone the next time you go shopping. Women tend to buy the same garment over and over again. Break out of your fashion box! Try pairing a tunic with leggings. Wear a fitted jacket. Wear a wrap dress with tights. Have fun!

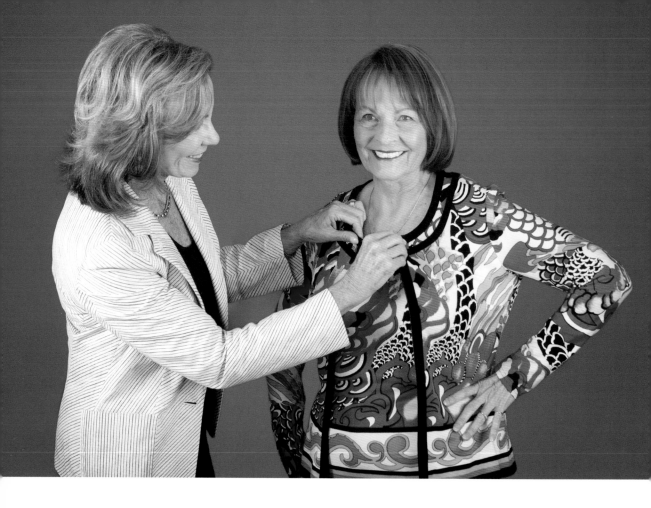

Whatever you do, make sure your clothes are the right fit. Fit and proportion are keys to looking current. So many women wear their pants too loose. Just because you are over fifty doesn't mean you aren't still a woman! Avoid pairing loose shirts with loose pants. It is a very unflattering look, even if you do have a model's body. If your top is a loose tunic, wear straight, fitted pants. If your pants are loose, wear a fitted top to enhance your curves. Fitted does not mean tight. If your clothes are too tight, they will draw attention to imperfections rather than flatter your figure. Look for clothes that mimic the lines of your body. A shirt or pants can fit without being restrictive.

Most outfits will come together if you accessorize correctly. The well-put-together woman is a pro at accessorizing. The right item can add just the right amount of pizzazz to an already polished look. Jewelry is the quintessential accessory. Gemstone stud earrings go with everything. Wear them by themselves during the day; pair them with a chunky necklace at night. Wear big earrings or a bright and colorful scarf to draw attention to your face. Be creative with scarf patterns or earring shapes. When it comes to shoes, wear whatever feminine style you like. Wear flats with skinny jeans. Wear wedge heels to add height while preserving comfort. Wear boots. These days, there are comfortable options in most any style. Wear whatever feels right—put your best foot forward.

I understand that sometimes finding clothes that you feel good in can be a challenge and you may feel like you can't find anything appropriate in stores. For example, it may be difficult to find shirts with sleeves in the summertime. Work around these obstacles. Buy the sleeveless shirt and layer a lightweight cardigan over it. **Don't get discouraged, and most important of all, don't give up.** Putting effort into the way you dress will make you feel good about yourself. Despite media bias, there is beauty in age—you just have to let it shine through. By investing a little time in your appearance, you will increase your self-confidence and therefore your well-being.

> The well-put-together woman is a pro at **ACCESSORIZING.**

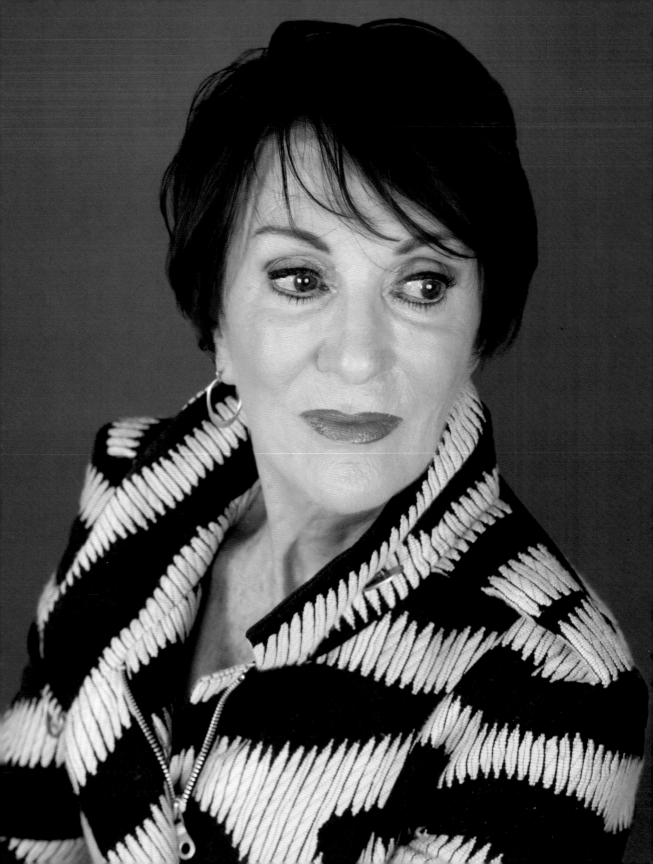

GIN

DUDE RANCH WRANGLER AND OUTDOORSWOMAN

Age: 74   Height: 5' 6"

Gin and her three brothers were reared by an athletic father and a musical mother. Her talented, encouraging parents urged their children to be involved in both physical and creative endeavors. Gin took up not only the cello but also the baritone horn. Her family had a summer cottage near a lake, so swimming was a natural choice for the adventurous girl.

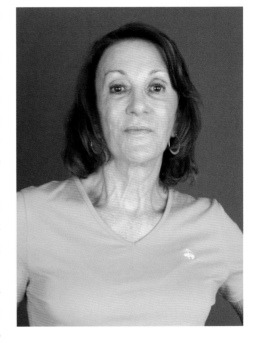

While in college, Gin was a store model for Saks Fifth Avenue and also took a job performing as a "mermaid" in the world's largest glassed-in swimming pool. Swimming wasn't her only athletic ability—she became interested in gymnastics, and even more interested in the young man who was her spotter on the uneven bars. They were married during the last semester of their senior year of college, and together they joined the very first Peace Corps class. The young couple was stationed in Ecuador, where Gin gave birth to her first son, became fluent in Spanish, taught at the local high school, and helped deliver babies in the municipal hospital.

After leaving Ecuador and returning to the United States, Gin worked as a swim coach and Spanish teacher and was blessed with two more children. After retirement, the happy couple moved to a small ski community in the Rocky Mountains, where her husband spent his final years. After her husband's death, some friends invited Gin to visit their guest ranch for a diversion. They knew that she loved horses, but little did they know that Gin would remain a wrangler on their dude ranch for the next ten years.

She now spends a lot of her time outdoors enjoying the snow and the mountains with her three children, twelve grandkids, and many guests. Her high energy keeps her hiking high-elevation routes and skiing the black-level trails near her home. When opportunities arise, Gin is always up for travel and adventure.

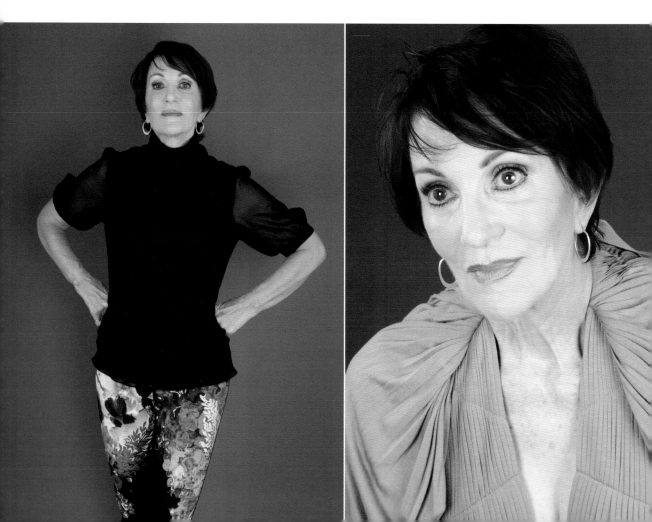

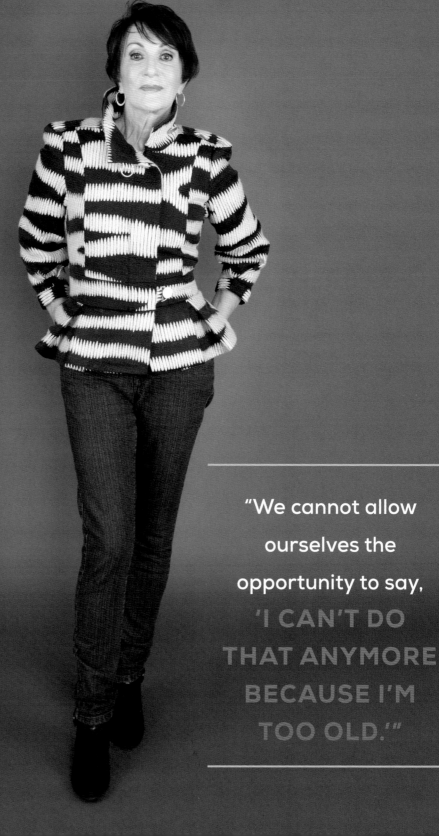

"We cannot allow ourselves the opportunity to say, **'I CAN'T DO THAT ANYMORE BECAUSE I'M TOO OLD.'**"

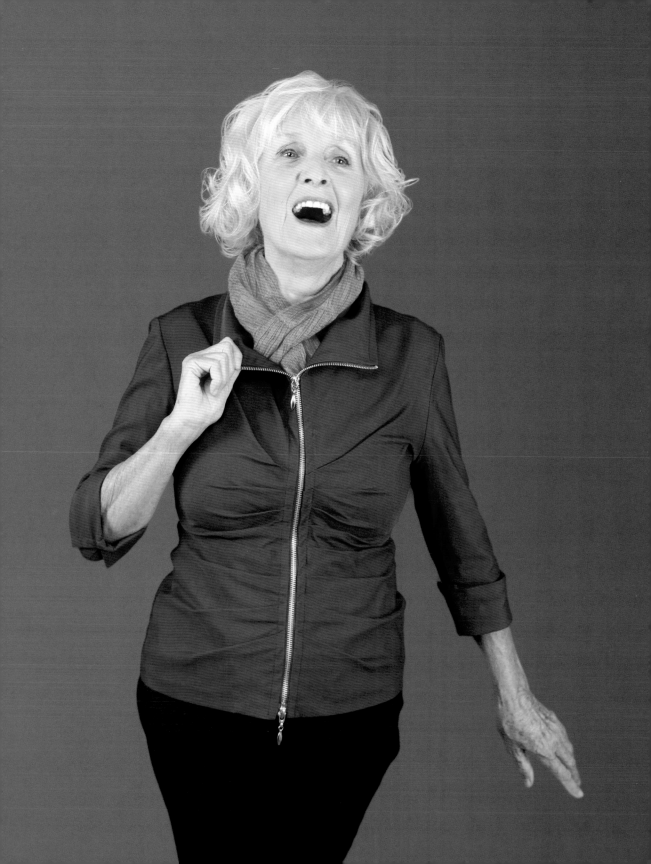

SUE

STUDENT OF HISTORY AND CULTURE

Age: 67   Height: 5' 3"

Sue's life has been driven by her fascination with history and linguistics, around which she has built her career and lifestyle. She loves to visit the places "where history happened."

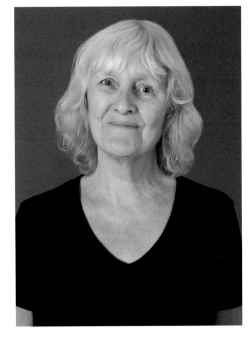

Sue was born in Manchester, UK, attended university in Wales, and studied in Paris. She feels lucky to have learned many languages in school and can converse in French, German, and Italian, making her travels around Europe that much easier. She has spent much of her time traveling independently, either by train or bus, staying in small guesthouses along the way. She loves to explore Roman and Greek antiquities, beautiful and off-the-beaten-path medieval towns, and both famous and local museums. Sue is eager to hear the stories of residents she encounters.

After completing her formal education, Sue began her teaching career in England, working in both London and Manchester. She then set off to Japan, where she taught English as a foreign language in

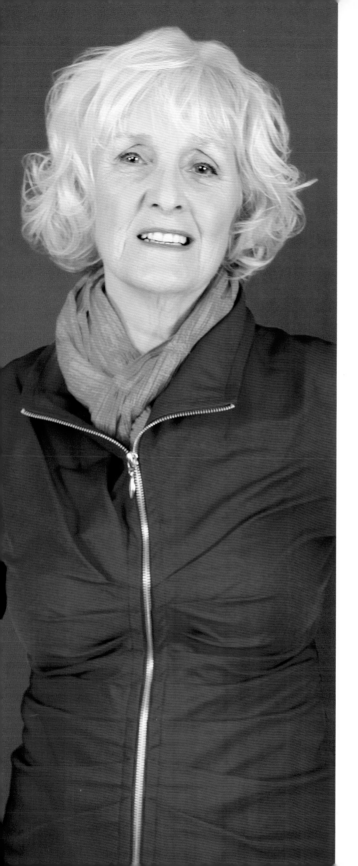

schools, universities, and businesses. There she immersed herself in the culture, learning Japanese, marrying a Japanese man, and having two children. In the late 1970s, Sue achieved a true traveler's coup, gaining access to China and Burma, which had been only recently opened to foreign travelers.

Sue moved back to London with her family in 1988, began catching up with the city's cultural activities, and took trips to Athens, Salonika, Istanbul, Sarajevo, and other less-visited places she had read about in literature and historical texts. While in London, Sue taught Japanese. In 2002, she relocated to Houston; since then she has taught at a local college, learned Spanish, and traveled throughout the United States, the Middle and Far East, Europe, and Central America, where she explores the spectacular natural settings and wildlife. As she thinks about retirement, South America is next on her travel agenda.

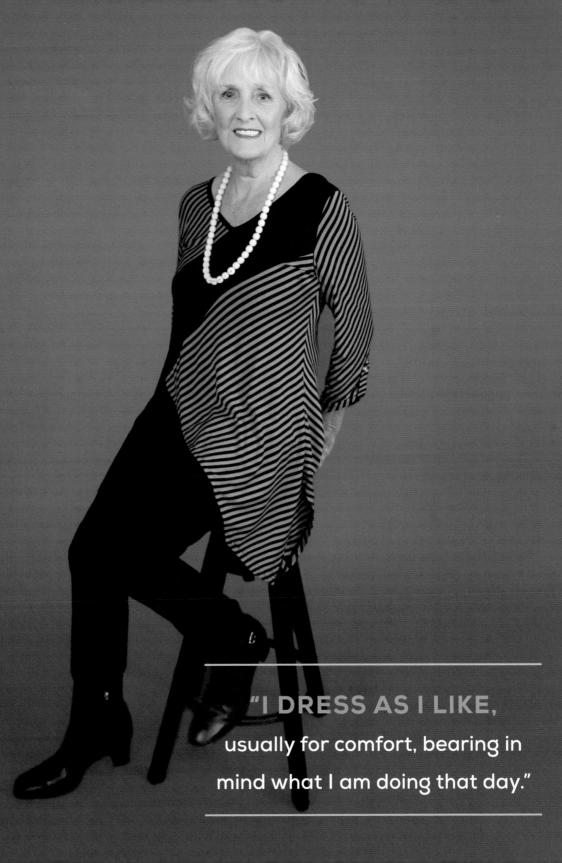

"I DRESS AS I LIKE, usually for comfort, bearing in mind what I am doing that day."

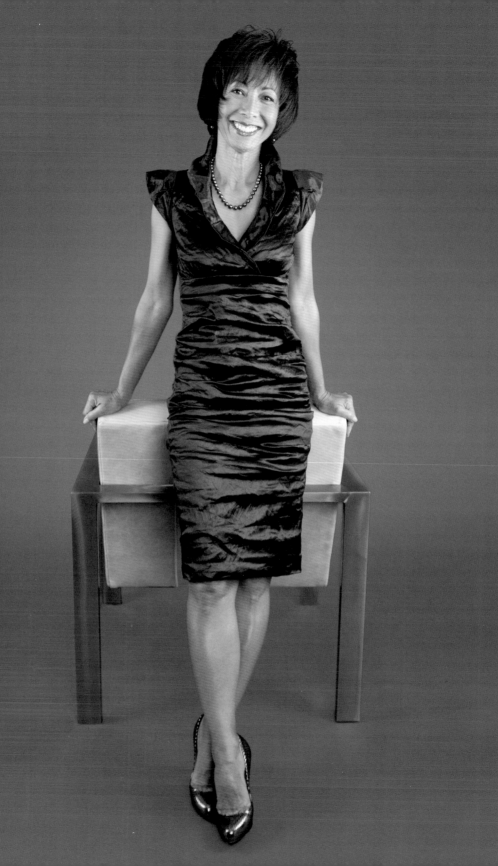

GERI

MARATHON RUNNER AND GENEROUS MENTOR

Age: 66   Height: 5' 2"

Geri loves staying active, and she likes for her days to begin with gardening, swimming, golfing, Pilates, biking, or any of the many sports she enjoys. But fifteen years ago, Geri couldn't run a quarter of a mile without huffing and puffing; when she was challenged to run a marathon, her response was, "I hate running; it's boring." Today Geri has completed marathons not only in all fifty states but also in Cozumel, Athens, Medoc, Paris, and Iceland. Her husband, Ron, often joins her, running half marathons and enjoying the beautiful golf courses around the world. Geri has made many friends in her travels and enjoys getting to know new people while she runs. Her encouraging and optimistic spirit is a welcome boost to anyone she encounters.

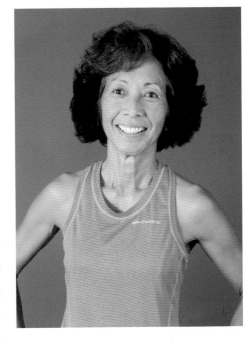

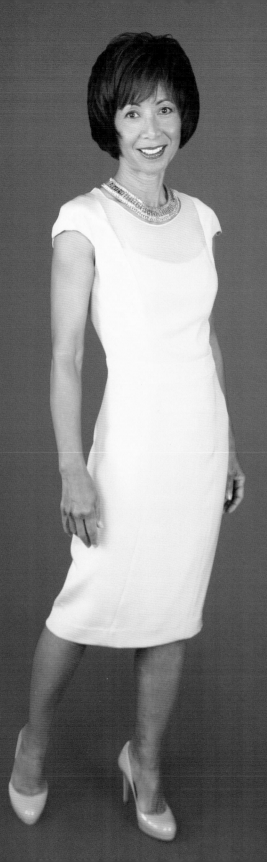

"Enjoy this chapter of your life by making time for friends and family, praising God for the blessings, and **CONSTANTLY TESTING YOUR LIMITS.**"

She is now participating in triathlons, which will allow her to give her knees a rest and to concentrate on total body conditioning. She notes that although she is a Hawaiian Islander, she doesn't enjoy swimming as much as running and biking, as swimming is not as social.

Geri now has a young granddaughter, Lina. They love to read and paint together, and Geri, or Tutu—"grandparent" in Hawaiian—is overjoyed to have Lina in her life. Another rewarding aspect of her life has been her call to go on short-term mission trips to Mexico and Guatemala. She helps out in her own community through a ministry designed to aid young mothers who seek stability. Geri serves as a proud mentor and companion, providing guidance and encouragement.

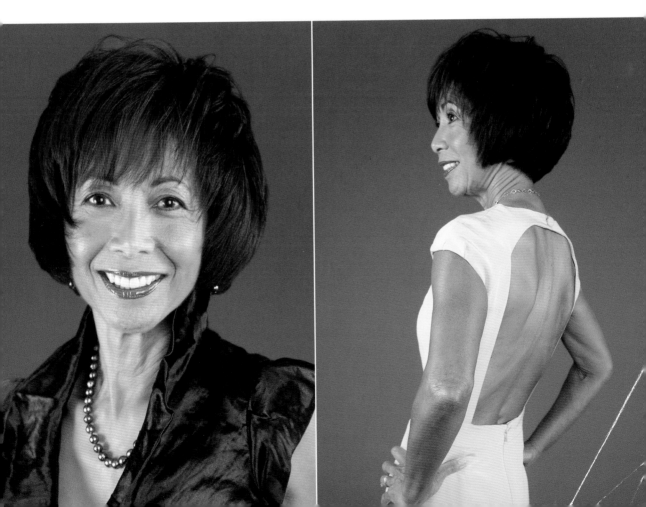

Hair-Styling Solutions

JOEL HOLLAND, MASTER HAIRSTYLIST

I have a vivid memory of my father, who had a very large hair salon in Las Vegas, styling twenty show-girls before a show. I can still see each woman with her hair in a roller set, sitting under a large, bubble-hooded hair dryer. When they were dry, each girl's hair would need excessive teasing and a lacquer of hair spray. The beauty industry has certainly changed dramatically in the thirty-six years I have been doing hair, but so much remains the same.

Making a woman feel beautiful is always my first and most important consideration. This has been the foundation of my career. Vidal Sassoon's trademark saying, "If you don't look good, we don't look

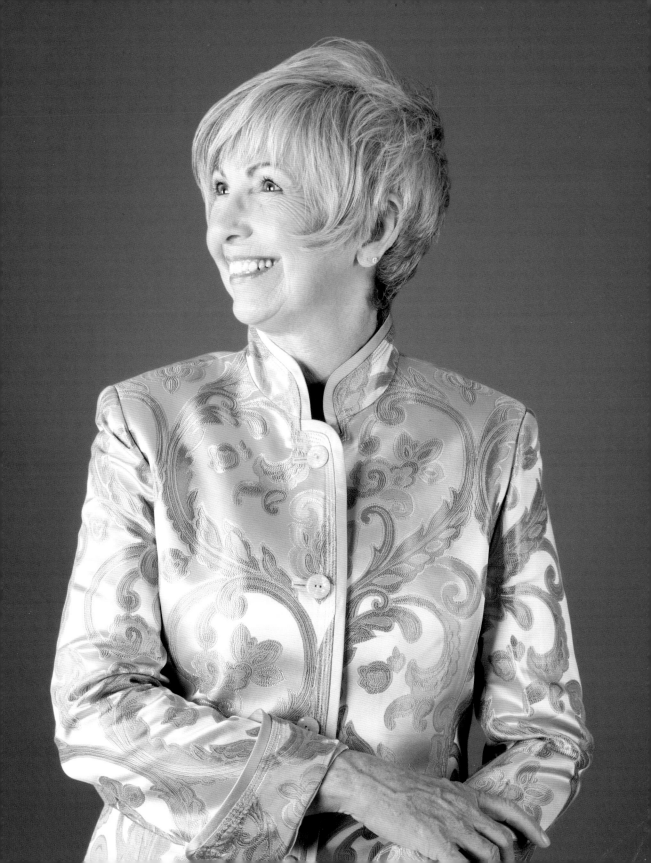

> Keep in mind, it takes the eyes **SEVENTY-TWO HOURS** to adjust to any change in appearance.

good," could not be truer. All women—no matter their age—want to feel beautiful. There used to be an unspoken rule that once a woman went gray or reached a certain age, she must get a permanent and cut her hair short. This is no longer the case, especially since products and dyes have changed and improved.

When working with a client, I take into account several details, including age, face shape, features, weight, height, and even lifestyle and career. There are no set rules—every woman presents a different combination of elements. So it is important and necessary to begin with a thorough consultation in order to achieve the best results and avoid a style that might not be appropriate for the client.

Common mistakes include choosing the wrong color or style or being unwilling to update a dated look. For you as a client, it is essential to seek out unbiased opinions and, if necessary, be willing to leave your beloved hairdresser in order to get a fresh opinion and look.

Hair Color

When hair begins to gray, it tends to lose its warmth and becomes more ash- or cool-toned, so adding warmth back into the color is necessary even if the client wishes to stay with her natural gray.

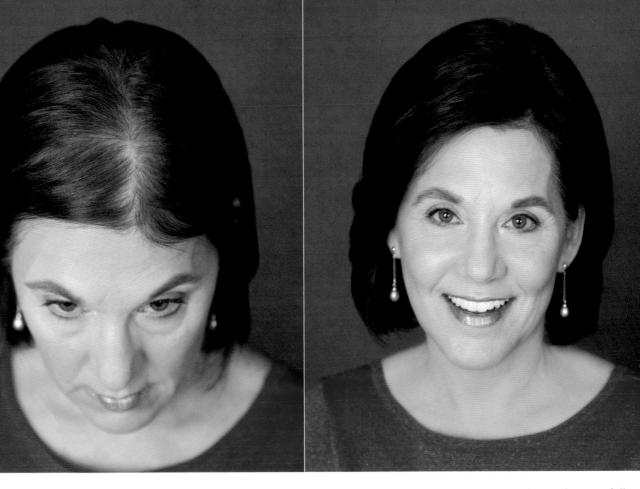

Like many women, Diane's hair is thinning.

Her hairstylist used a **topper** to make her style more full.

THINNING HAIR
Diane, 60

There are several options for thinning hair, including hair extensions or using a hairpiece. Consult your stylist for product recommendations.

To Cut or Not to Cut

Many older women will ask if they should cut their long hair short because of their age. For some women, short hair might be a great option. But for some, it's not a necessary step to update one's look. Talk to your stylist about the best cut—long, short, or in-between—for you.

Procedures

Advances such as keratin hair straightening, tints, dyes, and gloss treatments have made such salon procedures more accessible and more affordable.

Tools and Maintenance

A good stylist will offer a full explanation and tutorial on how to style your hair. Make sure you know which tools (brushes, blow-dryer, curling or flat iron) and methods are needed to get the desired result at home. With the innovations in home styling tools, you should need only a few minutes to achieve your favorite style.

It's important you use only the best hair care products on your aging hair. Although they can be expensive, their ingredient quality and concentration levels are higher.

Finally, proper ongoing maintenance is also key to keeping your look fresh. Plan to get your hair cut and colored every four to six weeks.

Remember, if you find yourself with a hairdresser who is unwilling to change or update your style, it may be time to look for a new one!

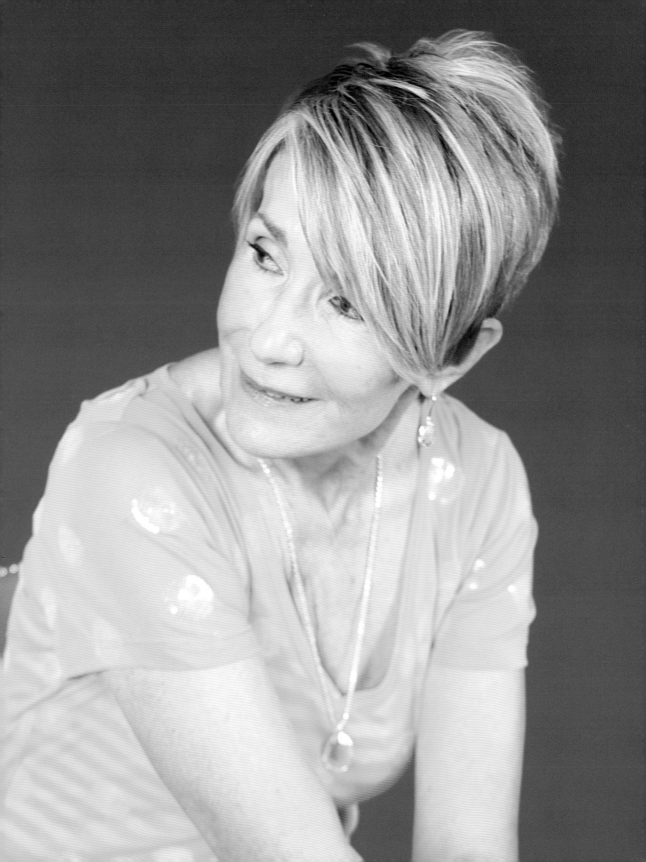

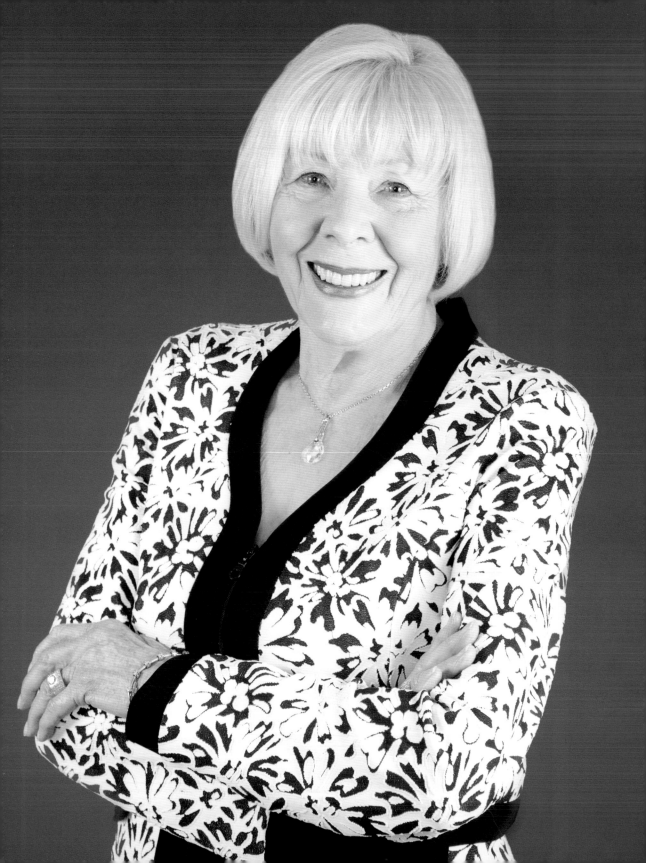

BARBARA

A NATURAL LEADER AND CURIOUS MIND

Age: 80   Height: 5' 5"

Barbara graduated from nursing school in Ohio as a registered nurse (RN) and became licensed in Connecticut; she was the first nurse from out of state to take her board exams. She was interested in psychiatric nursing and felt privileged to work at one of the best hospitals in the country. She and her husband settled down in Connecticut to raise two sons and a daughter. During her children's formative years, Barbara worked as a school nurse so that she could be home when her kids were there. She earned her bachelor of science at age fifty.

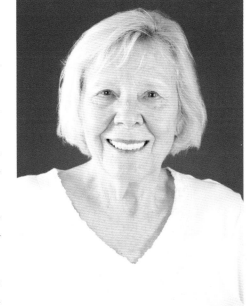

After her children were out of high school—and for the next fifteen years—Barbara worked as a certified travel counselor, one of the few with that credential in the business. She used her intellect and energy to book both business and leisure travel. Before retiring, she was a coordinator of trade shows, overseeing dealers, manufacturers, venues, entertainment, and more.

Barbara is an adventurous traveler. She has memories of seeing

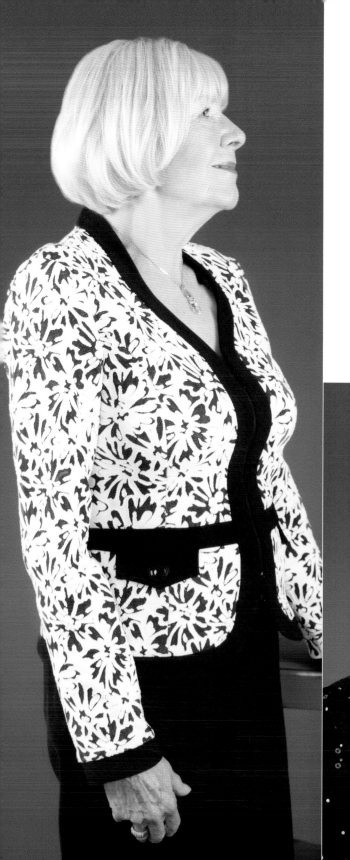

many of the world's wonders—not only as a tourist but also as a mother and grandmother visiting her children while they lived and worked abroad.

Now a widow, Barbara recognizes she must have people in her life. Her bridge game and organizational skills enliven the local bridge scene, and local college classes and lectures help satisfy her curious mind. Her first priority remains, and always will be, her children and their families, but she is sought after socially for her positive attitude.

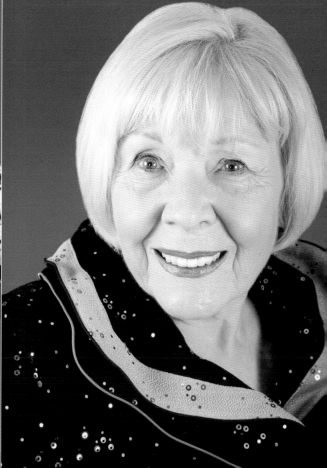

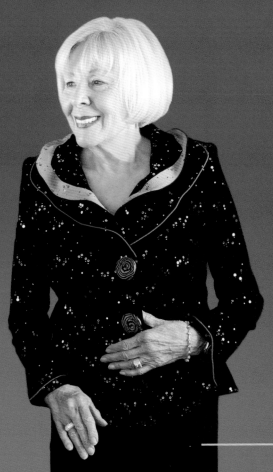

"THERE IS
LIFE AFTER
KIDS, TENNIS,
HUSBANDS,
AND CAREERS...
however short life is,
it does go on with
what one makes of it."

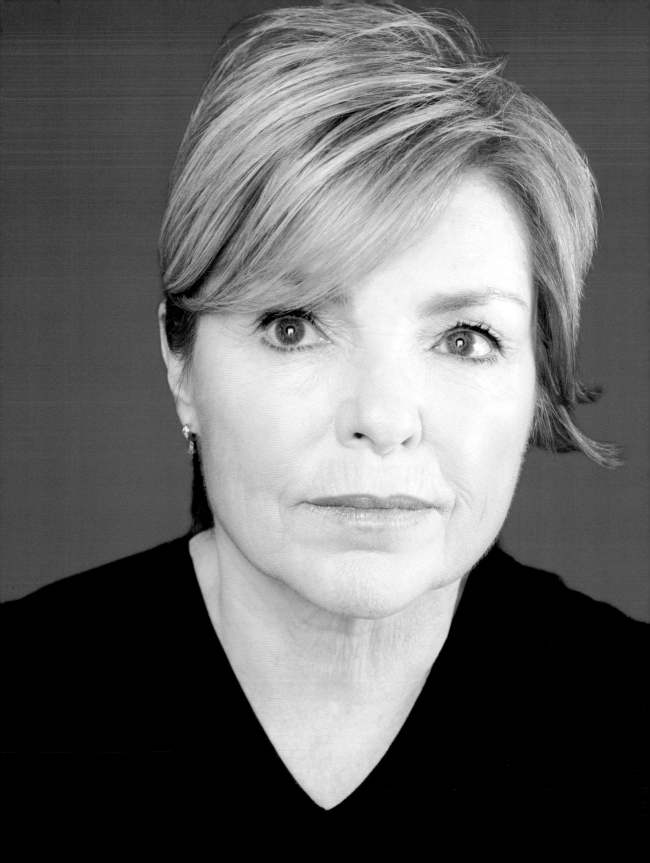

ANNE

SON'S MILITARY SERVICE GIVES HER STRENGTH

Age: 65   Height: 4' 10"

Anne is happy to be the mother of two wonderful sons and the wife of a supportive and encouraging husband. When her oldest son announced his desire to serve his country as an officer in the army, Anne wasn't sure she could handle the stress that would come with the knowledge that her son was risking his life. She admits that his four years of training at West Point did not prepare her for what lay ahead. The pageantry of the parades, the stately military balls, the traditions of the Army-Navy Game, and the grandeur of the graduation ceremony distracted her from the stark realization that her son would soon be at war. Seeing the camaraderie between her

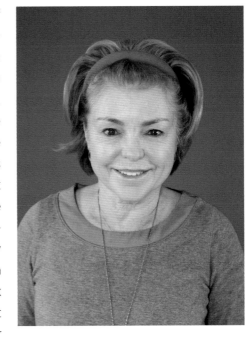

son and the other men in his company gave her a bit of solace on the day of his deployment. But as time went on, it was the support of her husband and fellowship with other military families that helped her to build the strength required to get through such uncertain times. Anne

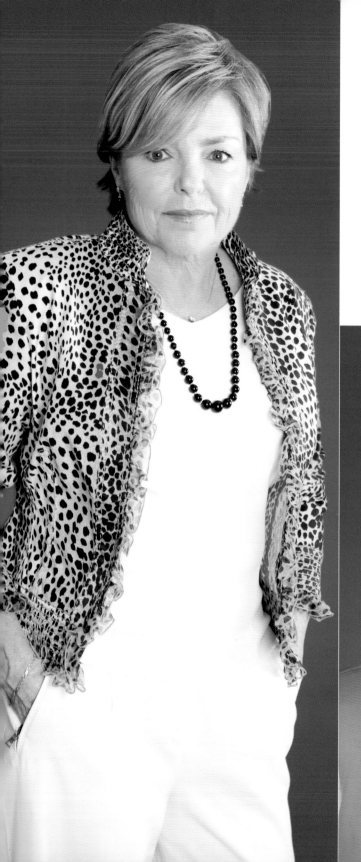

found comfort in the company of other military moms—no pretense was necessary when she was among those going through the same experience. They confided in each other and were able to freely voice their true feelings and fears. Her son is now a civilian and she can rest easy, but Anne will forever cherish the inner strength and faith that the experience forged in her.

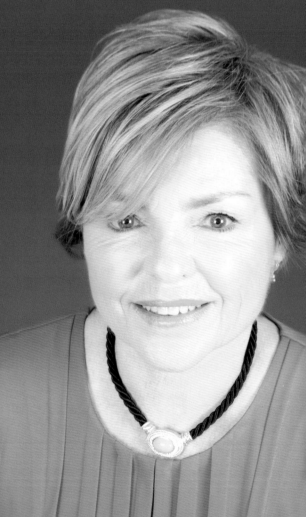

"One should always strive for what the Italians call *fare la bella figura*, which means to not only dress well but to **GIVE A GOOD IMPRESSION** and show that one is on top of every situation."

Exercise at Any Age

CLINT JOHNSON, MPT

Why Is Exercise Important for Seniors?

Millions of people exercise regularly to stay in shape, lose weight, or just feel better. It is well known that there are many benefits of being in a regular exercise routine. Exercise can make you feel better physically and emotionally. Regular exercise can increase your energy level and provide great stress relief. As we age, however, the benefits of exercise take on a whole new importance.

Our Aging Bodies

Our nation's population is aging. People are living longer and the baby boomers are increasing the senior population. It is becoming increasingly important for health-care workers to educate our senior population about the benefits of exercise. A regular exercise routine is essential to help seniors not only improve their quality of life but also continue to live safely on their own.

As we age, our bodies and physical abilities change. We lose muscle mass. Our muscle flexibility decreases and our joints become more rigid and susceptible to osteoarthritis. Our sense of balance can diminish, too, as a result of overall muscle weakness and physical changes that cause a shift in our center of gravity. Poor balance increases the risk of falling and fall-related injuries.

A regular exercise program developed for an individual's specific needs can improve functional strength and flexibility, which in turn reduces those risks. In fact, exercise can do many things to improve one's physical health. Studies have shown that regular physical activity can help reduce or stabilize blood pressure, improve symptoms of arthritis, and combat obesity and its associated conditions such as diabetes.

Exercising on a regular basis can also help people feel better mentally and emotionally. It can increase energy and help us deal with stress. For seniors, incorporating a regular fitness regime into daily life is particularly crucial. There are countless ways exercise can improve our quality of life as we age.

Starting Your Own Fitness Regimen

Many people can be apprehensive about starting such a regimen—some are intimidated by the mere thought of it. They may be concerned about a past injury or a potential one. Or they may not know exactly which exercises are best for them. This is where health-care professionals can play a vital role, by getting seniors started on the path to improving their health with exercise.

If you are nervous about beginning an exercise program, a good starting point is a visit to your primary care physician, who can assess your health status and advise you about any restrictions or guidelines. If you have functional limitations, your physician can refer you to a physical therapist. The therapist can assess those limitations and create an exercise program specifically tailored to your needs.

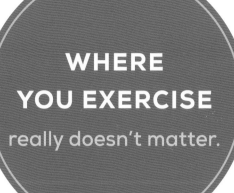

WHERE YOU EXERCISE really doesn't matter.

Four Types of Exercise

While many people work out at a local gym that has various types of equipment and even a swimming pool, other exercises are easily done in the comfort of your own home. Where you exercise really doesn't matter. Many workouts, whether aerobic or for flexibility, strengthening, or balance, are doable in any setting you choose. Performed properly and safely, all such routines benefit seniors.

Aerobic exercises—for example, walking, bike riding, swimming, dancing—are aimed at improving your cardiovascular fitness. You may want to start a program by simply walking. I also recommend pool exercises for seniors who have access to an indoor pool or gym with a pool. Water aerobics classes can be helpful both physically and mentally. Your body benefits from the resistance training and the aerobic training. And being in a class—water aerobics or any other kind—is social and creates camaraderie. It can help you feel better about yourself and motivate you to work harder.

Strengthening or **"resistance** training" exercises build muscle strength and muscle mass. You can perform them with resistive bands, light dumbbells, ankle weights, or even soup cans from your pantry,

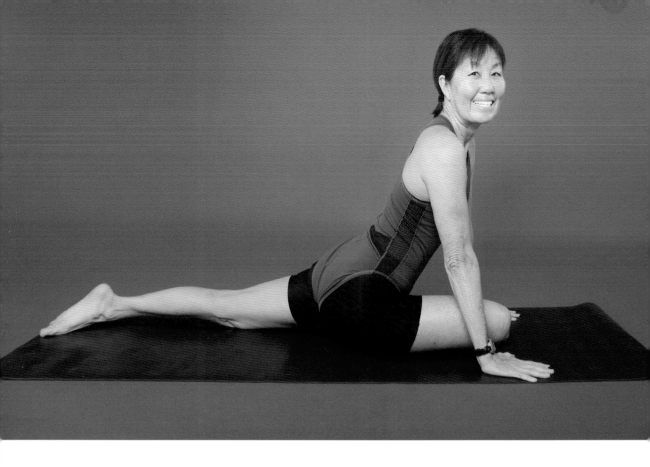

A good beginning schedule for embarking on an exercise program is three times a week.
MAKE IT PART OF YOUR ROUTINE.

which can be just as effective as the weight machines and equipment at a gym. If you choose to work out at a gym, I recommend completing an orientation with a gym employee or trainer before engaging in weight machine training.

Flexibility exercises focus on stretching legs, arms, and core. Maintaining good flexibility in your muscles and joints helps improve posture and balance and can reduce risk of falls.

Balance exercises are very important for seniors but can also be the most challenging exercises to do. They include standing on one leg, walking in a straight line (heel to toe), and marching in place. Consult a physical therapist or personal trainer to learn about more difficult balance exercises and make sure they are safe for you. Be sure you have supervision at first for any type of balance maneuver, to prevent falls and injuries.

> **DON'T FORGET** that fitness can be found even outside a planned exercise program.

Find Fitness All Around You

A good beginning schedule for embarking on an exercise program is three times a week. Make it part of your routine. Just remember to visit your physician before you begin.

Finally, don't forget that fitness can be found even outside a planned exercise program. Any form of activity (strolling in the mall, grocery shopping, walking a pet) can be beneficial. **What is most important is that you start moving your body—no matter what your age.**

Good luck!

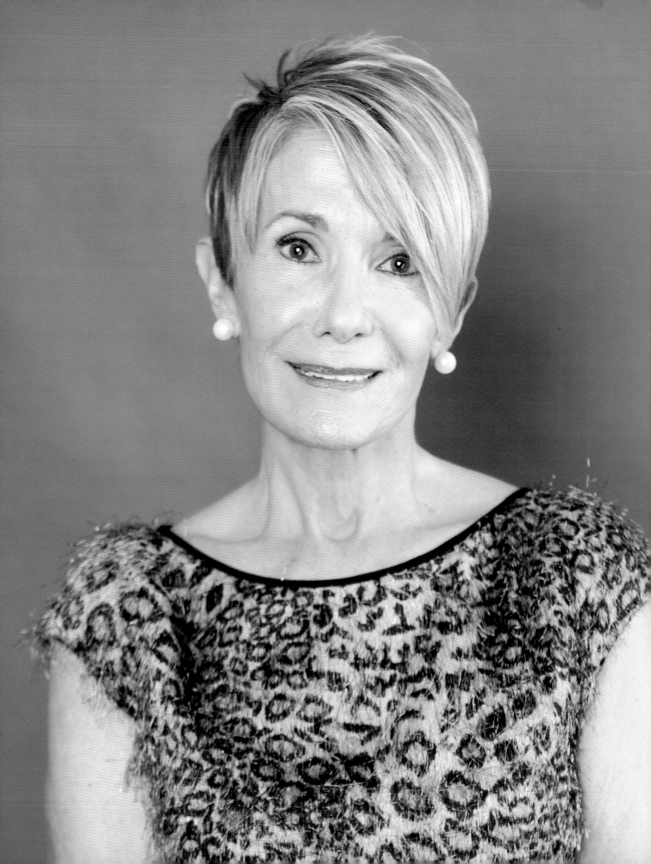

JANET

ADVENTUROUS TRAVELER AND GOOD FRIEND

Age: 69   Height: 5' 6"

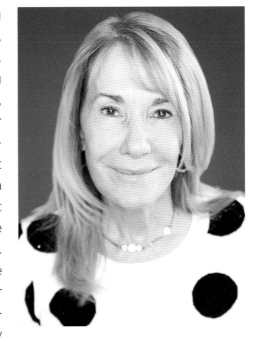

Janet is a firm believer in seizing the day. She has learned that at her age, there is no excuse to bypass opportunities. While she and her husband were sitting in a small room in Scottsdale, Arizona, begrudgingly listening to a sales pitch for a time-share as penance for taking a bargain golf trip, neither of them realized that this boring presentation would turn into a dream come true. Janet decided to invest in a time-share, which has changed the way she and her husband live their lives. It forces them to vacation. Janet's three sons had been eager to visit Ireland—their grandfather's place of birth—and the time-share gave the family the opportunity. They visited his town and farm, met relatives for the first time, and listened to stories. Her middle son was so enamored of Ireland that he obtained citizenship.

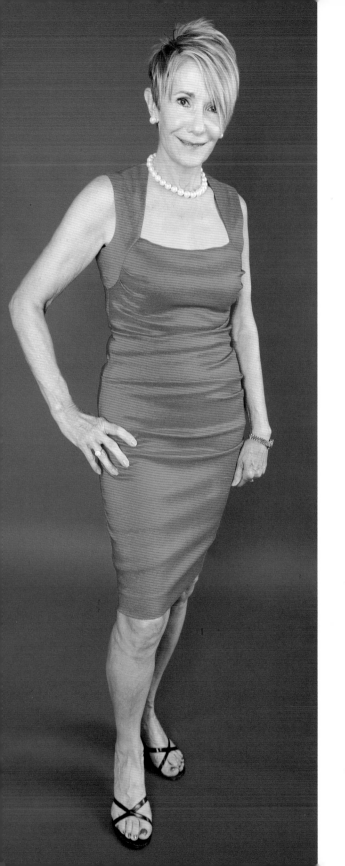

Janet's travels include adventures of all sorts. When the zip-lining instructor encouraged her group to "freestyle," Janet eagerly flipped over and crossed a Canadian creek upside down. At Atlantis resort in the Bahamas she swam with dolphins and barreled down every waterslide. In Kauai, Hawaii, she flew over the island in the front seat of a helicopter.

As her children have left home and started their own lives, friends have become a larger part of Janet's. A few years ago, she and a group of friends took a girls' trip to Galveston to celebrate ten years of friendship. They ended up being there the same weekend as a biker rally, but the ladies embraced the change of pace. During that trip, Janet got her first tattoo; no one, so far, has told her she'll be sorry about it "when she's older."

"As long as my health is good, I plan to continue **PUSHING THE ENVELOPE.**"

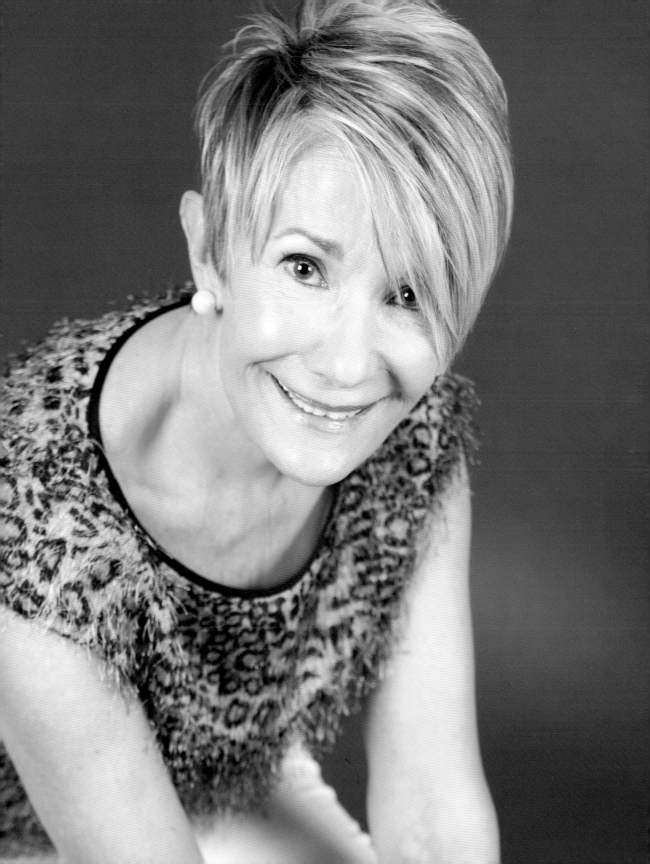

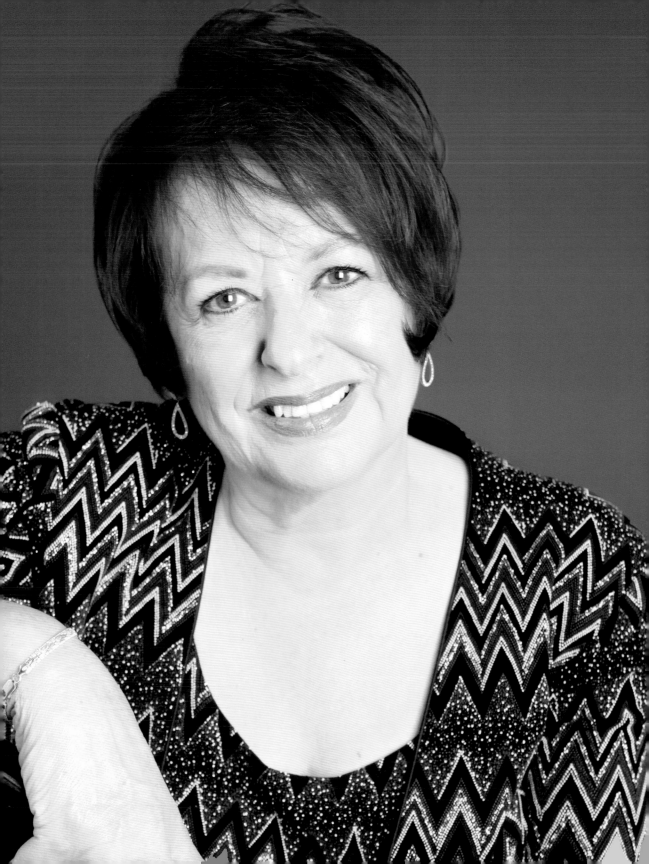

MARGARITA

CANCER SURVIVOR AND WOMAN OF FAITH

Age: 65   Height: 5' 5"

Margarita's faith has guided her through many of life's journeys, including her battle with cancer. Her journey to recovery has made her a stronger woman and renewed her soul. Maintaining a positive spirit and keeping a radiant smile on her face helps her stay focused on the joy that surrounds her.

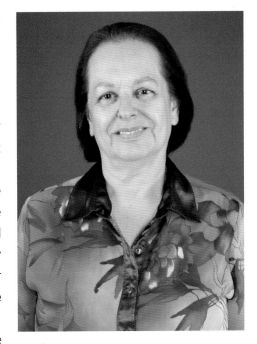

Margarita is a believer in taking life one day at a time. She makes certain to take time for daily prayer, asking God to bless her and her family. Margarita thanks the Lord every day for every breath and gives freely of her generous and caring nature; her positive outlook warms the lives of many.

Margarita is an independent single woman and is excited to have time to focus on herself at this stage in life. She loves to travel, but when she's at home spends much of her free time appreciating the arts—going to the theater, museums, and

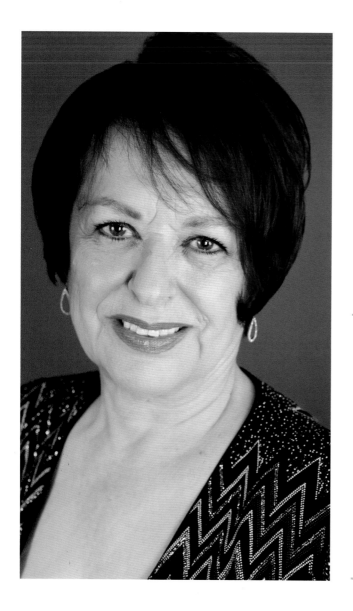

the symphony. She is active in various women's groups and participates in community outreach.

Margarita loves to follow fashion and takes pride in a polished and attractive look. She is content with who she is but thinks there is always room for improvement.

"There's nothing that can stop me from feeling pretty and stylish. I'M CONTENT WITH WHO I AM!"

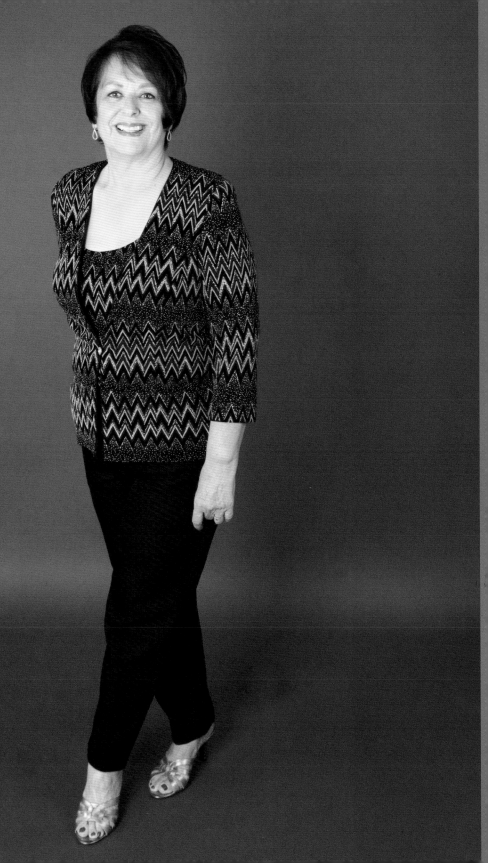

Facial Rejuvenation After Age Fifty

SABRINA A. LAHIRI, MD, FACS

BOARD CERTIFIED BY THE AMERICAN BOARD OF PLASTIC SURGERY

Facial rejuvenation has evolved rapidly over the past decade to keep pace with women's desire for a more youthful appearance. The practice has become more accepted and mainstream, creating opportunities to look more youthful and feel reinvigorated. Introduction of successful products and procedures has revolutionized the specialty of cosmetic facial rejuvenation. The role of the plastic surgeon has changed to include many different nonsurgical options for fighting facial aging. Effective treatments, both nonsurgical and surgical, are now available from both plastic surgeons and, increasingly, medical spas.

Skin Care Products and Procedures

Finding the right clinician is an important aspect of considering which cosmetic facial procedure to choose. I recommend that patients do their research on potential physicians or spas before making their selection. Seek out a board-certified plastic surgeon who is experienced in facial procedures. Or, if you are thinking about visiting a medical spa, make sure it has an on-site medical director who is well versed and qualified in cosmetic procedures. Lower price is rarely the best reason to pick a physician or facility.

Nonsurgical methods for facial rejuvenation, ranging from medical-grade skin care products to injectables, have swiftly gained popularity in recent years. The first step in restoring youth and vibrancy to your appearance is treating the skin with prescription products that are proven to help bring about a major change in skin quality. There are countless lines of so-called therapeutic products out there, so be sure to choose only those that are reviewed positively in the medical literature. Typically, over-the-counter and department store products are not as effective.

> **EFFECTIVE TREATMENTS,** both nonsurgical and surgical, are now available from both plastic surgeons and, increasingly, medical spas.

I often advise clients to consider one particular line of therapeutic skin care products called ZO Medical, which was founded by skin health guru Zein Obagi, MD. Products such as these, as prescribed by your clinician, restore skin's appearance by treating fine lines, large pores, dark spots, poor texture, and acne. Every patient who considers delving into facial rejuvenation should always have a solid home treatment regime in place. These products are the basis for beautiful results whether or not you choose to pursue a more intensive approach.

Chemical peeling has been a mainstay of noninvasive rejuvenation and a safe and effective treatment for skin imperfections since the 1950s. Peels, however, have evolved and improved over the years.

EVERY PATIENT
who considers delving into facial rejuvenation should always have a solid home treatment regime in place.

Today, most are performed in a medical spa setting under the supervision of a physician, who uses various formulations to target different skin conditions. Not only are chemical peels a good value but they also typically entail minimal discomfort and inconvenience. Patients peel for three to five days, a relatively brief downtime.

Even more than chemical peels, laser treatments have exploded onto the market in recent years. Choosing a qualified clinician is paramount, because the wide array of possible treatment types can certainly be confusing. Newer fractionated lasers—including the popular Fraxel and Pearl—are among many different brands available that are replacing full-face CO_2 laser resurfacing for treatment of wrinkles, pigmentation, and laxity. Intense pulse light treatments also improve texture and help minimize wrinkles and spots. This treatment, commonly called the "photofacial," has been proven over the years and is a mainstay in most aesthetic settings. A quality physician or medical spa can guide you to the correct treatment for you, laser or otherwise.

Some treatments, such as Thermage and Ultherapy, employ a specific type of device to treat facial laxity. These machines use radio frequency or ultrasonic energy to tighten the deep soft tissue of the face. Benefits include firmer-looking, smoother skin and better definition around the jaw-line and neck. Although the procedure is effective, results appear over a matter of months. A single treatment stimulates new natural collagen production for up to six months; depending on your skin condition, results can last for years. Practitioners have performed more than one million Thermage procedures worldwide; the procedure is safe and can target the areas that are most bothersome. Yet these devices will have little overall effect on patients with too much facial laxity.

Injectables

More invasive treatments for facial rejuvenation are also widely available, starting with injectables that range from neurotoxins to fillers. Botox, Dysport, and Xeomin—three popular variants on the botulism toxin—temporarily weaken the action of localized muscles that creates wrinkles on the face. These products are most effective for the inevitable "11" creases that appear between the eyebrows on the forehead as we age.

Traditional fillers, such as hyaluronic acid, come in liquid or gel form. The products plump up areas of the face to "fill in" lines, wrinkles, and creases. Your clinician can prescribe any one of several effective fillers, including Restylane, Perlane, Juvederm, and Radiesse, to ease lines around the mouth, elevate marionette lines, and plump up lips. All these methods have long-lasting (typically up to nine months) but not permanent results.

Injectables have entered new territory with an exciting approach that actually stimulates collagen production. Rather than a quick fix, it is a subtle process that offers longer-term results—up to two years. Sculptra Aesthetic (injectable poly-L-lactic acid) is the first facial injectable that encourages the body to replace lost collagen and reinforce the skin's structure from within the deep dermis to gradually fill in facial wrinkles, from the shallow to the deep. As the skin absorbs the microparticles of this product, a collagen framework is created that can rejuvenate the entire face, creating an overall youthful appearance. The mildly uncomfortable treatments are performed in three different sessions, each taking approximately forty-five minutes in an office setting. In a major clinical study published in the *Journal of Cosmetic Dermatology*, 80 percent of the patients treated with Sculptra Aesthetic were satisfied with their results.

Platelet-rich plasma injections are another evolving treatment for facial rejuvenation. Referred to as the "vampire face-lift," this procedure involves drawing a patient's blood and injecting the plasma portion back into the face. The dermal injection stimulates the production of a collagen scaffold, releases growth factors, and attracts, proliferates, and differentiates stem cells. All these activities help the skin and tissue transform back to their youthful appearance, with improved skin texture and volume. Using the patient's own blood encourages tissue regeneration, helps ensure that the process is nonallergenic, and eliminates the risk of transmissible diseases.

Typically one to three treatments are recommended, each performed in the office in about one hour with minimal discomfort, but more may be needed for better results. Patients start to see improvement after three weeks, and results usually last more than a year. There are more than 25,000 scientific papers on platelet-rich plasma and, to date, no data has revealed any adverse side effects. All age groups can benefit, although the procedure is not recommended for smokers or people with chronic disease or cancer.

Surgery

If a patient has an abundance of loose skin and sagging deep tissue, nonsurgical treatments will not improve the aging face. For those who desire more results, surgical treatment has been the mainstay. **The most common rejuvenation surgeries include eyelid lifts, face-lifts, and neck contouring.** Blepharoplasty, otherwise known as an eyelid lift, treats slack or sagging skin on both upper and lower eyelids. Excess fatty deposits that appear as puffiness or bags are removed. Eyelid surgery is usually performed on adult men and women who have healthy facial tissue and muscles and realistic goals for improvement. The procedure is performed under sedation or general anesthesia. Your more youthful appearance will appear gradually as

IT IS IMPORTANT for a prospective patient to do research on the quality of her chosen clinician.

swelling and bruising subside over several weeks, though it may take up to a year for incision lines to fade.

Technically known as rhytidectomy, a face-lift is a surgical procedure to treat the visible signs of aging in the face and neck. It is recommended when minimally invasive procedures will not be effective. Several areas can be addressed: sagging in the midface, jowls created by loss of muscle tone in the lower face, loose skin and excess fat under the chin and jaw, and deep creases along the nose extending to the corner of the mouth. A face-lift does not change your fundamental appearance and cannot stop the aging process. This is a highly individualized procedure, and you should do it for yourself, for your own purposes—not to fulfill someone else's desire. It may take several months for swelling to fully dissipate and up to six months for incision lines to fade. A healthy, nonsmoking lifestyle will help extend the results.

Choosing the Right Option

There are many options for facial rejuvenation that are available in many settings. It is important for a prospective patient to do research on the quality of her chosen clinician, whether it is a cosmetic surgeon or a nurse injector. Most qualified plastic surgeons will offer numerous options for rejuvenation, from noninvasive methods to surgical interventions. The surgeon will customize the treatment to each individual patient. Any one of these procedures can lead to wonderful results that can leave you feeling happier as you age gracefully.

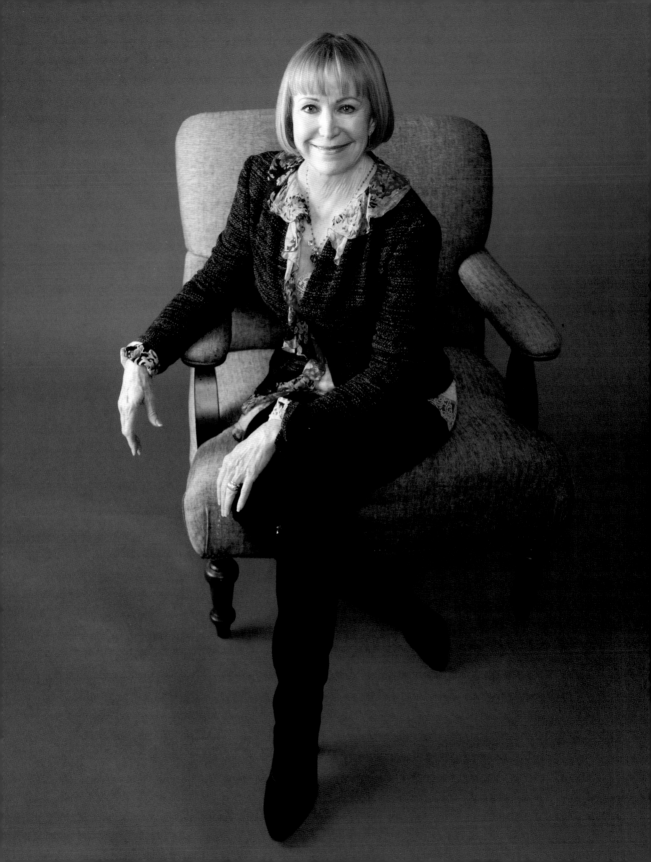

WENDY

FASHION MAVEN AND POSITIVE SPIRIT

Age: 68   Height: 5' 7"

Wendy grew up in Southern California and has loved the arts since an early age. Yet her original career path led her to the USC School of Dentistry. Her affinity for the arts and fondness for fashion were relegated to leisure time. Part-time modeling kept her in touch with her aesthetic side; Wendy believes you always have a better day when you look your best. She added a creative spin to her work attire by wearing cashmere sweaters, sleek slacks, and high heels with her lab coat rather than the usual scrubs and nurse's shoes. Wendy soon realized that spicing up her wardrobe wouldn't make her like her job any more in the long run.

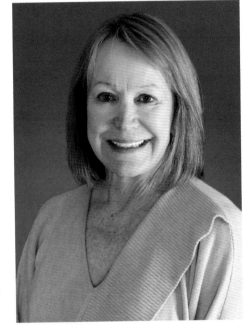

After twenty years as a dental hygienist, she transitioned into a career more in line with her artistic bent: she became co-owner of a women's boutique in California, gaining experience in buying, retail merchandising, and the harsh realities of meeting a bottom line. The contacts she made as a shop owner helped her

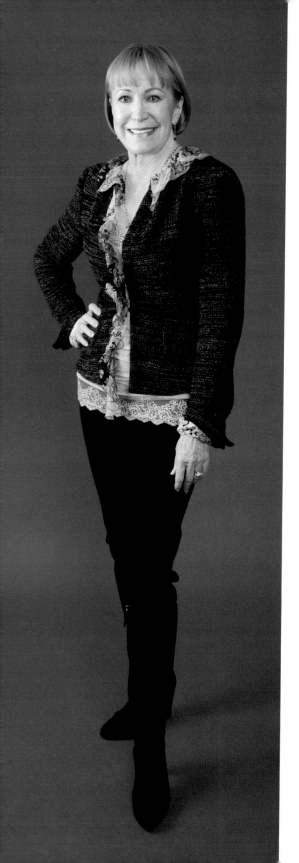

advance in the wholesale/retail industry, first in jewelry, then in ready-to-wear and Parisian haute couture.

From youthful modeling at I. Magnin in Beverly Hills to serving as national North America sales director for Christian Lacroix, Wendy did manage to weave her love of color, pattern, texture, and unique detail into everyday life. She was also fortunate to work with an artist and fashion designer from Thailand who produced exquisite silk fabrics in rich and vibrant patterns and hues. The commercialization of art to meet the demands of the real world posed challenges she'd known about as a girl but now fully embraced as a grown-up.

After many years of traveling the world and enjoying her work with creative and artistic people in fast-paced work environments, Wendy is retired from the fashion business. She appreciates the simplicity of a life without sales quotas, market share demands, and delivery deadlines. Her supportive husband, friends, and charity pursuits are now what fuel her zest for life, and she makes sure to embrace life's positives.

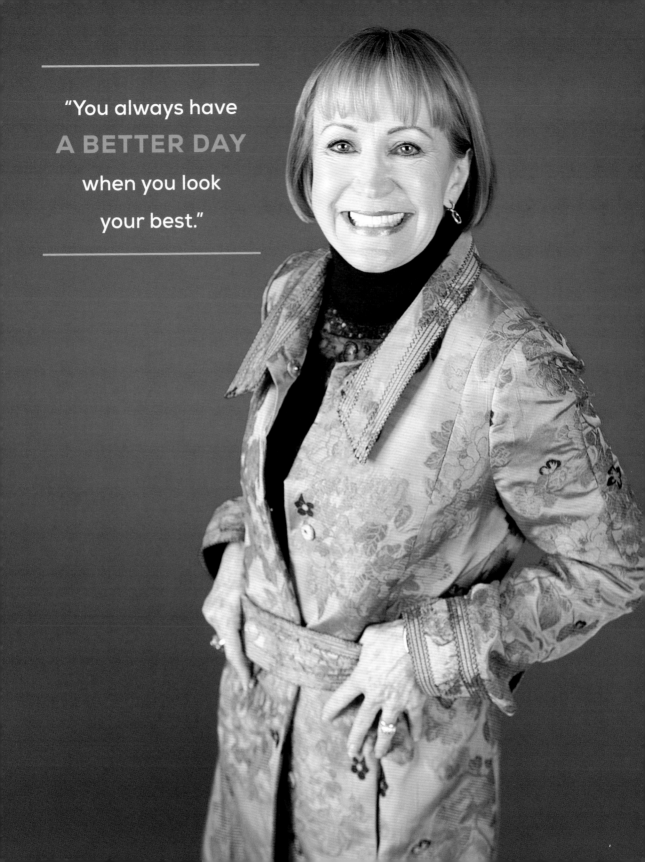

"You always have **A BETTER DAY** when you look your best."

MARGARET

FAITHFUL CHRISTIAN HELPER

Age: 61   Height: 5' 8"

Margaret was born in Uganda. She is the second-oldest child of eighteen brothers and sisters in a polygamous family. One of the happiest days of her life came when she married her husband, Patrick. But her happiness was short-lived—two days later her brother Peter was senselessly murdered by a rebel army. The pain this created opened her eyes to the prevalence of violence in this world.

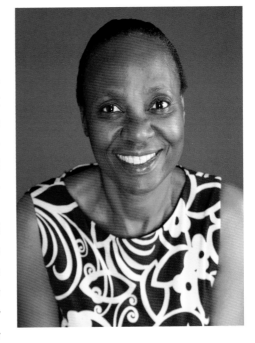

Margaret began a journey to understand why people must die. She was struggling to understand why a loving God would allow so much pain to occur. She wanted clarity to remove the animosity she carried in her heart. She found that clarity and was happy in her life as a Christian. But when war broke out in the Congo, Margaret felt that simply having strong beliefs wasn't good enough.

As refugees sought shelter in Uganda she learned a new way of life from them. These people had turned their suffering into a way to serve others. They traveled from village to village lifting the spirits of

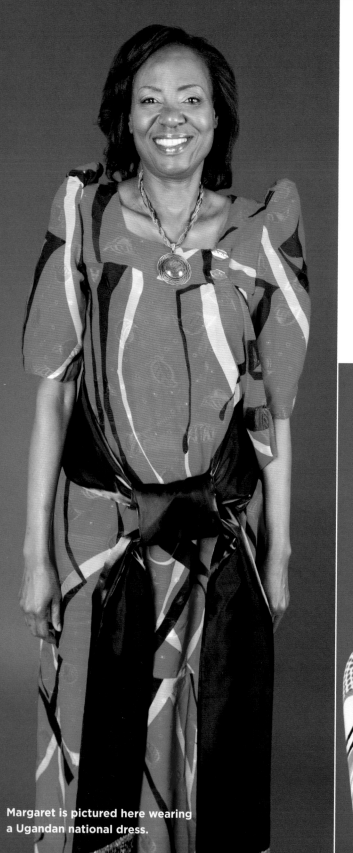

those in their path. Their example inspired Margaret to serve others more fully. She now devotes seventy hours a month to mentoring. She says her wealth is measured by the joy others derive from the hope they receive. She also feels it is important to remember to take time out for oneself to bring self-awareness, rejuvenation, and peace.

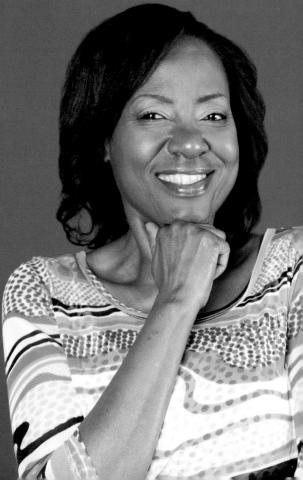

Margaret is pictured here wearing a Ugandan national dress.

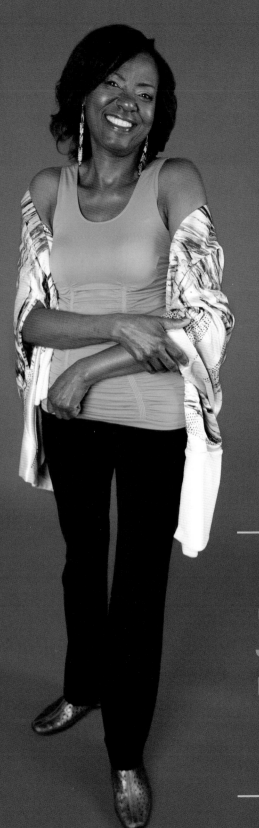

"My wealth is measured by the **JOY OTHERS EXPERIENCE** from the hope they receive."

Can You Hear Me Now?

SCOTT MARQUARDT, DOCTOR OF AUDIOLOGY

I would be surprised if anyone reading this has not come in contact with someone with hearing loss. It is at the top of the list of chronic health-care issues in the United States. Yet this issue is overlooked and ignored. My hope is to give you a brief overview of the hearing loss statistics in this country, along with an explanation of what causes hearing loss and the negative effects of untreated hearing loss. I also offer important tips for purchasing hearing aids and insights on technology advances that can make better hearing a reality.

Causes and Consequences

Hearing loss affects 10 percent of the entire US population. This comes to roughly thirty-four million people. When we look at the older age categories (above age sixty), the percentage increases dramatically. It is not hard to understand why there is a greater chance of hearing loss for a sixty-year-old than for a forty-year-old. You might think this is true simply because hearing loss is part of "getting old." Actually, we now think hearing loss can be attributed in most cases to noise exposure or a medical condition.

Harmful noise can come from obvious sources such as firing guns or work in a factory. Less obvious, however, are the normal noises we hear in everyday life: lawn mowers, television, phones, music, traffic sounds, and many more. These noises take a toll over the years and may ultimately result in hearing loss. Less common causes include medical conditions such as ear infections, wax impactions, diabetes, autoimmune disorders, and Ménières disease; medications and cancer treatments can also impair hearing. Some changes in neural processing do occur naturally and are related to the aging process; the transfer of information from the ear to the brain does slow down over time, which will certainly affect hearing, especially in noisy environments or groups.

Regardless of the cause, untreated hearing loss carries with it some very serious consequences. **Research has recently shown a link between hearing loss and dementia, Alzheimer's, depression, isolation, lower wages at work, and reduced sexual satisfaction.** Any one of these issues can negatively affect your retirement years.

Detection and Treatment

As is true with many other medical issues, early detection and treatment can be the key to maintaining optimal auditory function and health. Many people with hearing loss ignore the symptoms for years

> Depriving the brain of **AUDITORY STIMULATION** can cause the brain to "rewire" itself, making it difficult to adapt to treatment later.

before seeking help. Waiting too long before being diagnosed is a significant factor affecting treatment success. The results of untreated hearing loss can be likened to a person who sits in a chair and never gets out of it. Over time, the muscles you need in order to stand and walk begin to atrophy. It is the same with hearing. Depriving the brain of auditory stimulation can cause the brain to "rewire" itself, making it difficult to adapt to treatment later. Thankfully the brain can, in many cases, relearn to hear. The longer someone waits, however, the longer this learning process can take.

Treatment for hearing loss is becoming increasingly effective. **Depending on the type and degree of hearing loss, treatment can include surgery, hearing aids, and other assistive listening devices.** The first step is to undergo a hearing test with a doctor of audiology, who will be the person to guide you through any treatment that ensues. Finding the right hearing health-care professional is an important factor in patient happiness. Doctors of audiology have the highest level of training in testing hearing and providing amplification solutions. A great resource for finding an audiologist in your area is:

www.audiology.org

If a test indicates hearing loss, the next step is deciding which solution is right for you. Your audiologist may refer you to an ear, nose, and throat physician (otolaryngologist) to pursue reasons for hearing-related symptoms or to discuss surgery options, if appropriate. The audiologist may also discuss hearing aids that are appropriate for your lifestyle and needs. Each year, hearing aid technology is improving. We now have wearable devices that are not only extremely effective but also cosmetically acceptable. Some can connect with ease to cell phones, television, public sound systems (at church, for example), and MP3 players.

Hearing Care and Products

With ten thousand baby boomers each day turning sixty-five, many businesses have recognized an opportunity to make money from this population. Some insurance companies are even creating their own websites for hearing aid sales. Thankfully, in many states this practice is illegal. Online sales provide a product, but the sellers often are unconcerned about the satisfaction of the patient. As with any medical procedure, the most important component of the treatment is the medical professional with whom you have formed a relationship. There is no substitute for a highly trained, highly professional, and caring audiologist.

Now that you are older, I encourage you to be careful in choosing the right care and products to promote good hearing. Be proactive about removing your name from unwanted mailing lists, and do research when you receive offers for "too good to be true" discounts. Getting fitted with a hearing aid, like all health care, is not an event; it is a process. Make sure you feel you can trust the professional to be there for you during the full process of regaining your hearing.

> **THERE IS NO SUBSTITUTE** for a highly trained, highly professional, and caring audiologist.

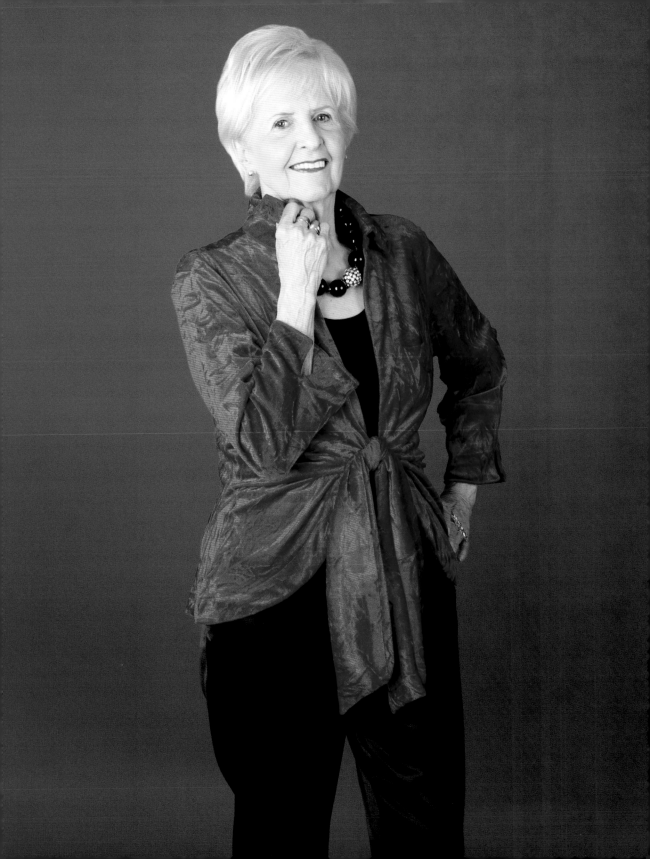

MARIE

CHANTEUSE AND TIMELESS BEAUTY

Age: 87   Height: 5' 4"

Marie has led a glamorous life. She has sung in nightclubs, modeled, and at age twenty-two won an Esther Williams Bathing Beauty contest. After attending school and working as both a secretary and model she married, at age twenty-nine, and had two children, whom she later reared as a single mother.

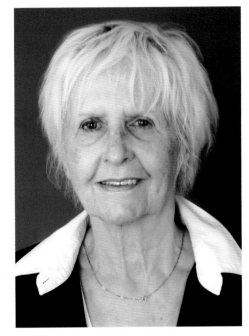

These days Marie still enjoys singing as well as art, painting, piano, exercise, and reading. She visits her local senior center almost every day, participating in bingo, art classes, and exercise. Marie is no longer able to drive, and though that makes life difficult, she still manages to remain active in her community—living proof that a senior center can be a social mainstay. She is well liked, generous, and an active friend to many others at the center.

Marie has an impeccable beauty routine. She takes great care to protect her skin from the sun and is often seen wearing a hat—even inside! A stunning woman, she has kept herself that way with regimens she initiated as a young woman.

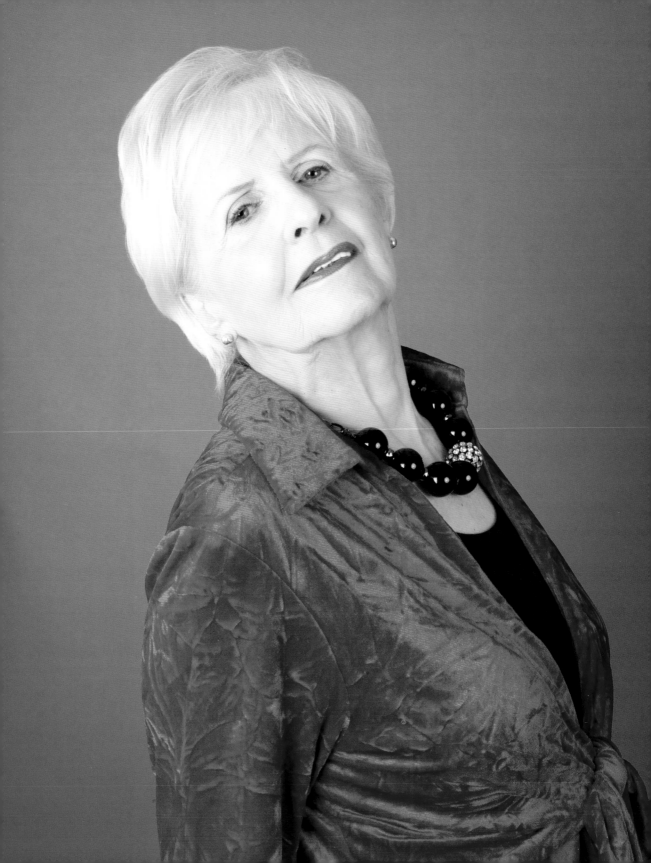

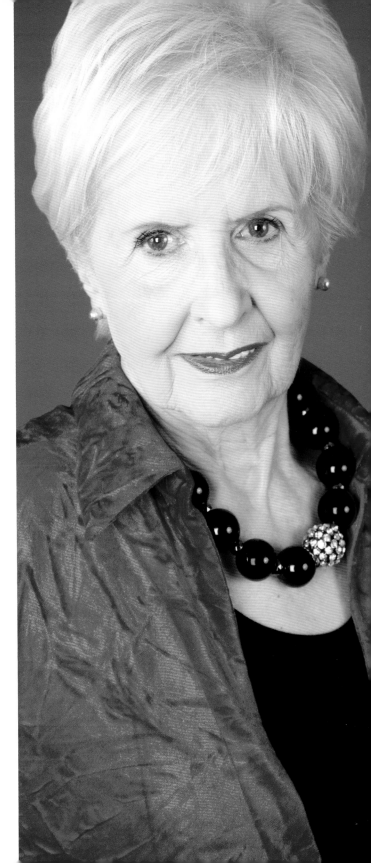

"**NOTHING MAKES A WOMAN MORE BEAUTIFUL**

than the belief that she is beautiful."

–Sophia Loren

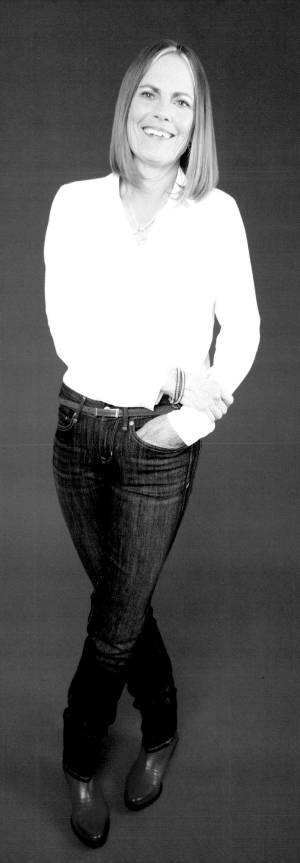

MAGGIE

ENTERPRISING HUMANITARIAN

Age: 67   Height: 5' 6"

In her youth, Maggie's nature led her to question the injustice in life. During her college years, both Vietnam and civil rights were on the forefront. Maggie graduated with a degree in social work, and as a college senior she married her best friend, Wally. They had four children and have lived everywhere from Germany and France to Texas and Colorado. While living in New York, Maggie found a way to combine her interests by becoming a social worker in a nursing home. In Paris she studied at Le Cordon Bleu, and in Chicago she went back to school and received a certification in early childhood education. In Houston, Maggie provided grief counseling and patient home care for a hospice.

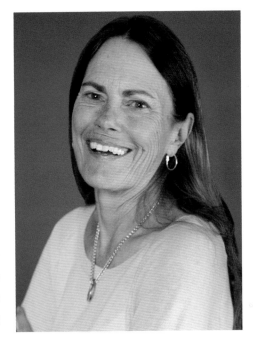

Maggie and her husband had long desired to move to Colorado. When Wally became ill, they realized that life was too short to hold off on following your dreams. So the empty nesters were off to Breckenridge, where Maggie found her voice and her passion. She became involved with a church-related safe place for young people seeking jobs and

"Our hope and dream was to **MAKE A DIFFERENCE** in the lives of people, families, and children in rural, remote villages."

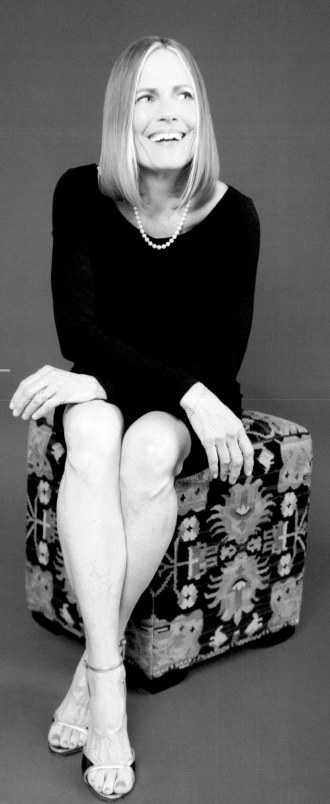

other resources to help with their daily lives. She also joined a church outreach group and traveled annually to Honduras. But she wasn't satisfied helping out only once a year and longed to establish a program that benefits people year-round. With her humanitarian non-profit Summit in Honduras, she aims to make a difference in the lives of families and children through medical and educational outreach.

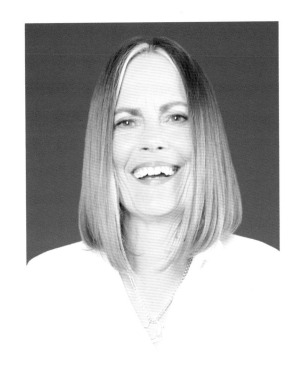

Maggie reflects on the years since the organization's founding: There are "tales to be told and mistakes that have been made, but we have done no harm, learned from our mistakes, and have definitely made a difference." In partnership with other organizations, Summit in Honduras has built three schools and rehabbed two others. It has also undertaken a major water project with the help of Rotary, partnered with Manos Amigos clinic to bring medical care and training to villages, and begun a partnership with the children's home Amigos de Jesus.

When working with a village needing a school or helping with a civic project, Summit in Honduras assists in fund-raising and also provides, most important of all, support for achieving success. The aim is that projects endure and can be sustained over time, even after construction is complete. The ultimate goal is to help and change lives, so that lives are not defined by poverty, but filled with hope and the tools for a better future.

Maggie had the extraordinary experience of meeting and spending some time with Mother Teresa while working in a soup kitchen with the Sisters of Charity in Chicago. She writes of the experience, "Mother Teresa has always been my hero and I believe in her words—that **'not all of us can do great things, but we can do small things with great love.'"** Maggie's own compassion radiates in everything she does.

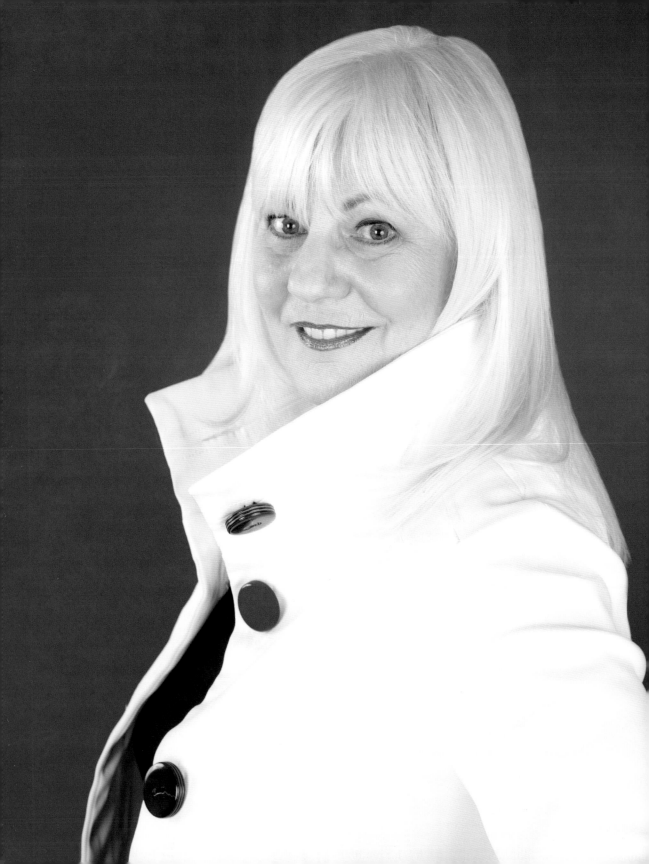

SUE

ARTIST, MUSICIAN, AND EDUCATOR

Age: 72   Height: 5' 3"

A retired special needs teacher with a master's degree in special education, Sue taught for twenty-seven years in Florida and Texas. She worked with children with physical, mental, and emotional disabilities. She found her career to be not only rewarding but also a great creative outlet.

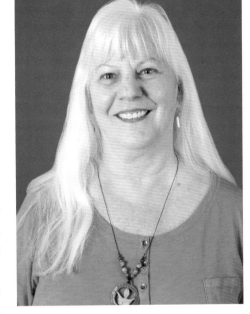

Sue has always enjoyed art and over the years has dabbled in many varieties of artistic media, including painting, drawing, and basket weaving. But after taking a ceramics class, she was hooked. Upon retiring in 2008, she set up a small home studio and has become an accomplished ceramics artist.

Another passion for her is music. Sue sang in choirs in school and played the piano as a child but did not actively pursue music until almost ten years ago when she joined the folk choir at her church, singing and occasionally playing the violin, an instrument she has recently learned. Soon after, she joined a band that is now recording an album. Between the two groups she gives at least four performances a month.

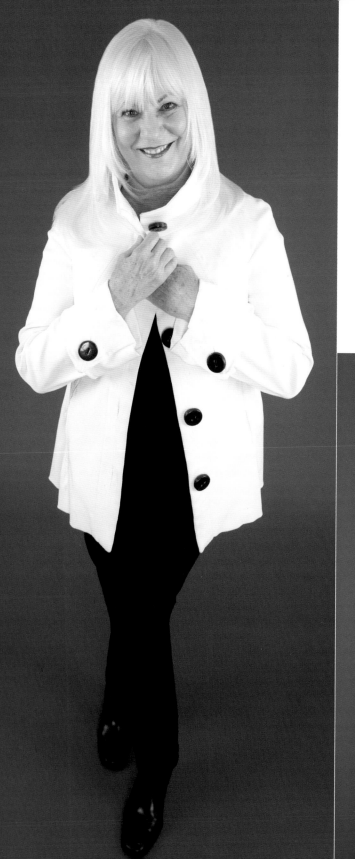

Aside from artistic endeavors, Sue enjoys gardening, reading, films, travel, and bird watching. Her two dogs keep her company, and she has a daughter who is planning to move to Texas soon. In her dress she typically gravitates toward casual, bohemian style, but she also loves to get glammed up for performances. Although her schedule is full and rewarding, Sue is always ready to try new things.

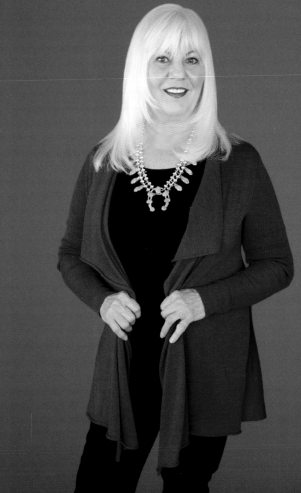

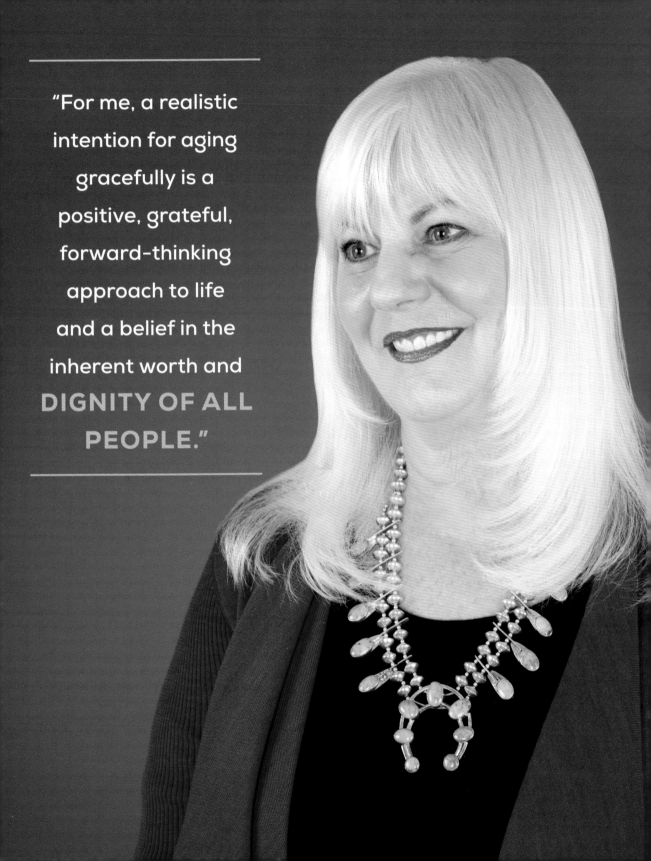

"For me, a realistic intention for aging gracefully is a positive, grateful, forward-thinking approach to life and a belief in the inherent worth and **DIGNITY OF ALL PEOPLE.**"

Skin Care and Makeup

MELISSA McKINNEY, MAKEUP ARTIST

The art of applying makeup shouldn't be scary, at any age. So let's take an inventory of what is and isn't in your makeup bag and in your skin care repertoire. When you're adjusting to a new and perhaps less demanding schedule, it's natural to become more relaxed about your make-up routine and to let go of some beauty rituals. The demands of the weekday have slowed. Seize this opportunity to kick-start your life with new makeup perfectly suited to your skin and your lifestyle. A woman who wants to make a fresh start is in for a renewing experience. Products are fun to buy and experiment with, but they can accumulate and overwhelm you with

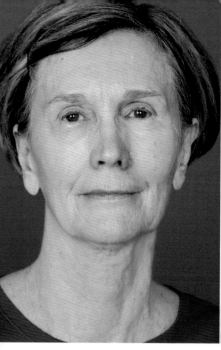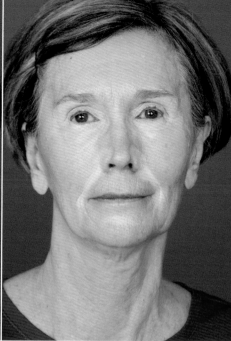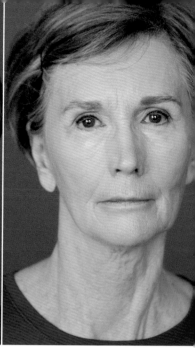

MAKEUP FOR THE MATURE WOMAN
Karen, 73

Karen has beautifully sculpted high cheekbones and deep-set eyes. **To prepare her face for makeup,** Melissa moisturized her skin and allowed it to absorb the moisturizer. If you choose to apply primer, now is the time to do so.

Apply concealer. This is your opportunity to make any "corrections" to your skin. Melissa applied an opaque, cream concealer to Karen's eyelids, as well as in the half-moon under her eyes and along the sides of her nose into her smile lines.

Melissa chose a light mineral **foundation** to cover and blend the concealer and even Karen's skin tone. Tinted moisturizer is another great type of foundation.

Melissa enhanced Karen's brows with powder using an eyebrow brush to apply and blend, accentuating the arch of the brow. A soft pencil is another good option for brows.

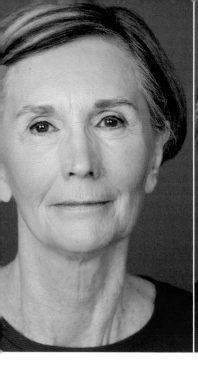
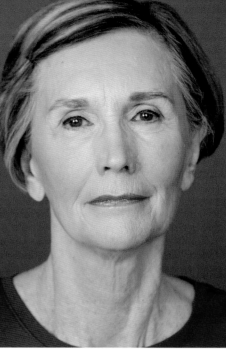
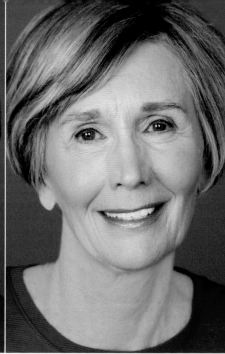

Melissa applied a **soft vanilla eye shadow** to Karen's brow bone, just under the arch of the brow. She shaded the eyelid with a light taupe shade and contoured the outer corner of the eye with a soft chocolate shadow. Melissa used a navy eyeliner pencil to line Karen's eyes and applied two coats of brownish black mascara.

Melissa applied a **rose blush** to the apples of Karen's cheeks, brushing upward at a slight angle into the temple area. She also lightly applied blush near the hairline and at the base of the chin. This brightens and accentuates Karen's face.

Melissa lined Karen's lips with a **light coral lip liner** and filled them in with a complementary shade of lipstick, enhancing her smile.

SEIZE THIS OPPORTUNITY
to kick-start your life with new makeup perfectly suited to your skin and your lifestyle.

choices. Once you know what works best for your skin, it's time to clean out your makeup bag, purchase a few must-have products, and get started with your new regimen.

Begin by finding an aesthetician to analyze your skin and focus on what you might want to correct or conceal. Although once-a-month facials may not be in the budget, your aesthetician can help you establish which cleanser, toner, and moisturizer will work for you and which special treatments, like exfoliants and masks, can improve your skin tone and texture. Equipped with your new knowledge, you can give yourself facials at home. A common mistake women make in their skin care is not keeping up with facial hair removal. Waxing is not the only choice; threading and laser hair removal have become popular techniques as well.

Find a trusted adviser, shop carefully, and **MOST OF ALL, BE BRAVE!**

Seek out a makeup artist for pointers on refreshing your techniques. Sign up for a makeup lesson, typically a one- or one-and-a-half-hour personal consultation; as you become comfortable with your new skills, you can learn additional tricks in subsequent artist visits.

While a consultation can provide specific, personalized suggestions as to color palette and the like, here are some general rules to follow when you're shopping for cosmetics. Avoid any product with a shimmer or pearl finish, as they can age the eyes and skin. Find a hydrating concealer that is one shade lighter than your skin tone. When choosing foundation or tinted moisturizer, select one that blends into your skin color. Test the foundation on your jawline, never on your hand, to ensure a good color match. As our skin ages, powder can become drying and can also settle into fine lines; use it only when really necessary. A triple-milled, translucent mineral powder is a good option if your T-zone gets a bit shiny. Using blush is important to highlight the cheeks, enhance bone structure, and add a healthy flush of color; fresh pink and peach tones lend a natural-looking glow. Bronzers can also help contour and provide flattering shape to the face.

Filling in and setting the eyebrows is vital for showcasing the eyes. A brow powder that blends with your hair color creates a soft effect; a pencil in that same color will give you more precise definition. Set the brows with a clear or tinted gel. **Eye shadows** in light, clean colors, such as a matte vanilla, highlight the brow bone. Apply a soft peach or rosy hue on your eyelids, and finish with a sweep of sable brown or gray in the crease. Blending your eye shadow colors is a must to prevent a paint-by-number look. **Eyeliner application** can be tricky for women who wear glasses. Invest in a magnifying mirror—it will become indispensable! An easy approach for those with shaky hands or less-than-perfect technique: Use a flat or angled brush to apply a dark eye shadow along the lash line. Dark brown, navy, or gray is a good choice and will enhance the eyes rather than make them appear small and tired. **Lashes** are always a concern for women; we want them to be thick and full, much like they were in our youth. You might try lash-growing serums, thickening primers, or volumizing mascaras to enhance your eyelashes. Applying mascara to the bottom lashes first helps keep you from getting mascara speckles on your lower lids.

A hydrating substance containing vitamin E will keep the lips moisturized; apply it at the beginning of the makeup process so it can be absorbed. **Lip color** is a personal preference. Many women prefer pink and peach, but anyone can wear red and rose tones too, as long as they are the right ones for your skin tone. Try mixing different lip colors to create your own color!

Remember, it's fun to reinvent yourself, and makeup is one way to be experimental in the comfort of your home. Find a trusted adviser, shop carefully, and most of all, be brave!

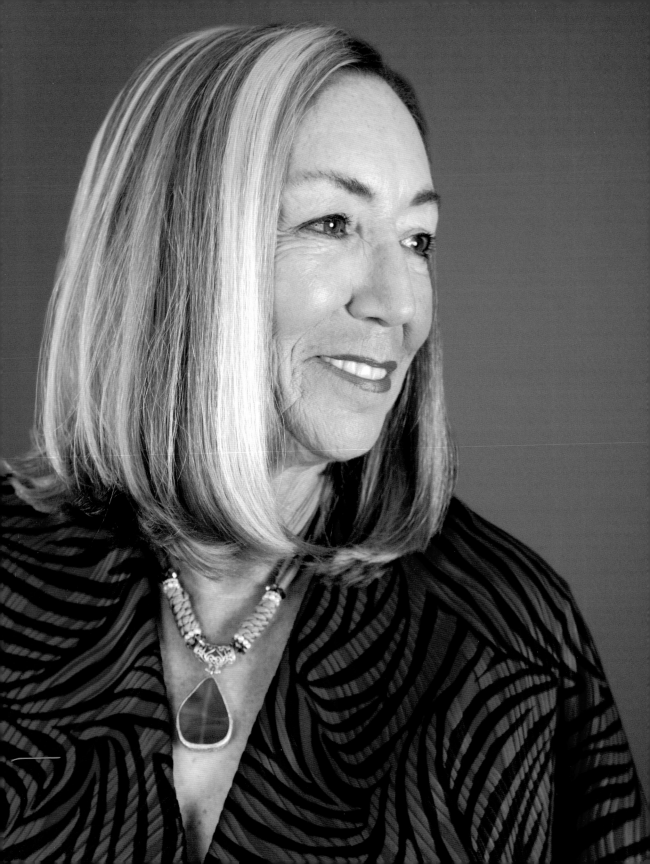

JANE

ENGINEER AND ENVIRONMENTALIST

Age: 67   Height: 5' 10"

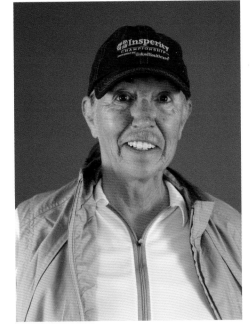

Jane was born on Maxwell Air Force Base in Montgomery, Alabama, where her mother and father were both pilots serving in World War II. She grew up in Bucks County, Pennsylvania, on a small but active farm where she developed a love and respect for nature and its creatures. She feels lucky to have attended a prep school, the Shipley School, in Bryn Mawr, Pennsylvania. Einstein once said education "is not the learning of many facts but the training of the mind to think"; that is precisely the sort of education Jane received at Shipley.

She went on to Lake Forest College in Illinois. Her ambition was to be an engineer, but at the time employers were still not inclined to hire women in male-dominated fields. After graduating, she moved to New York, where she began work as a file clerk at Texaco; during that time she taught herself computer science, becoming a systems engineer. She was selected to develop computer applications for her fast-growing company. Jane became an engineer after all!

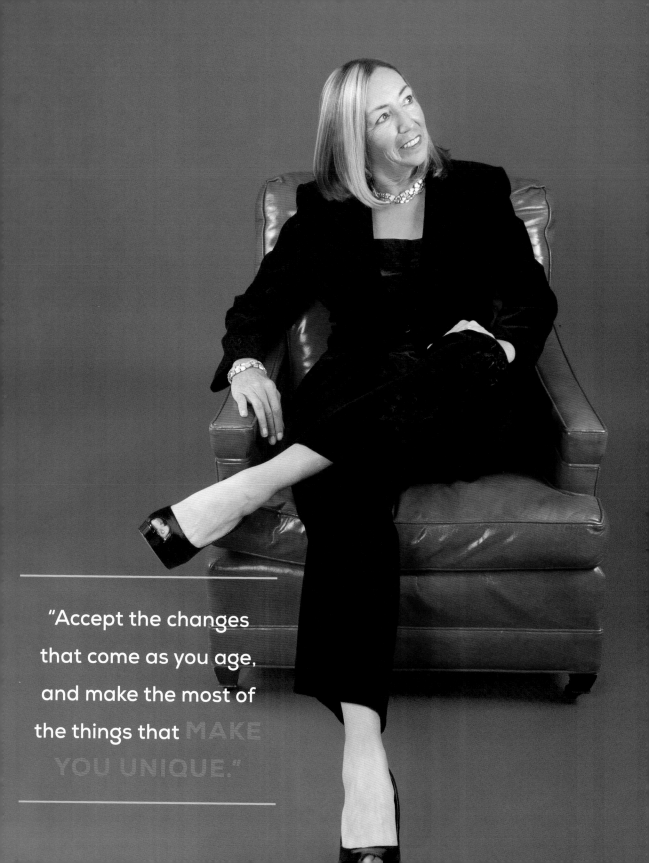

"Accept the changes that come as you age, and make the most of the things that MAKE YOU UNIQUE."

Jane retired in 2003 from Shell—which had bought her division from Texaco—as one of the top 10 percent of female earners in the country. She now enjoys card games, playing golf, spending time with her grandchildren, and restoring furniture. She and her husband moved to a beautiful area of Texas shortly before they retired. They now feel blessed to enjoy living in a place where there is a respect for and appreciation of the natural environment.

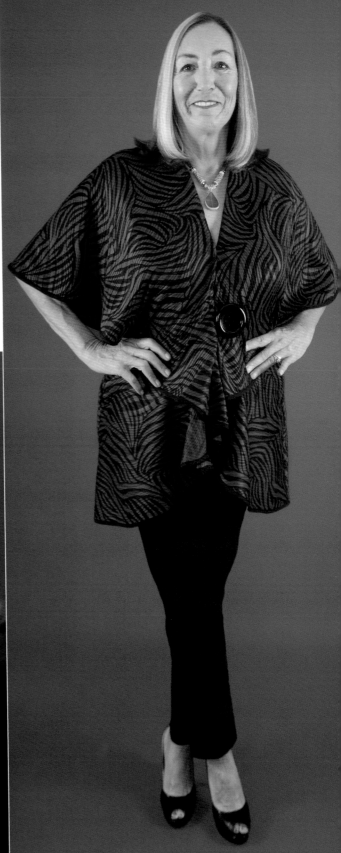

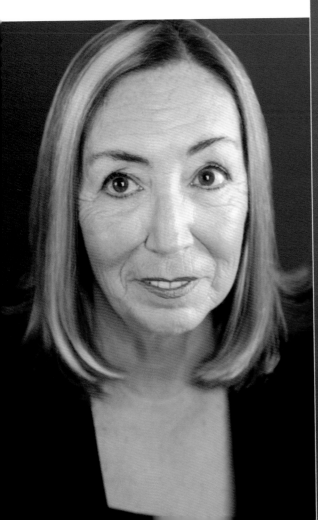

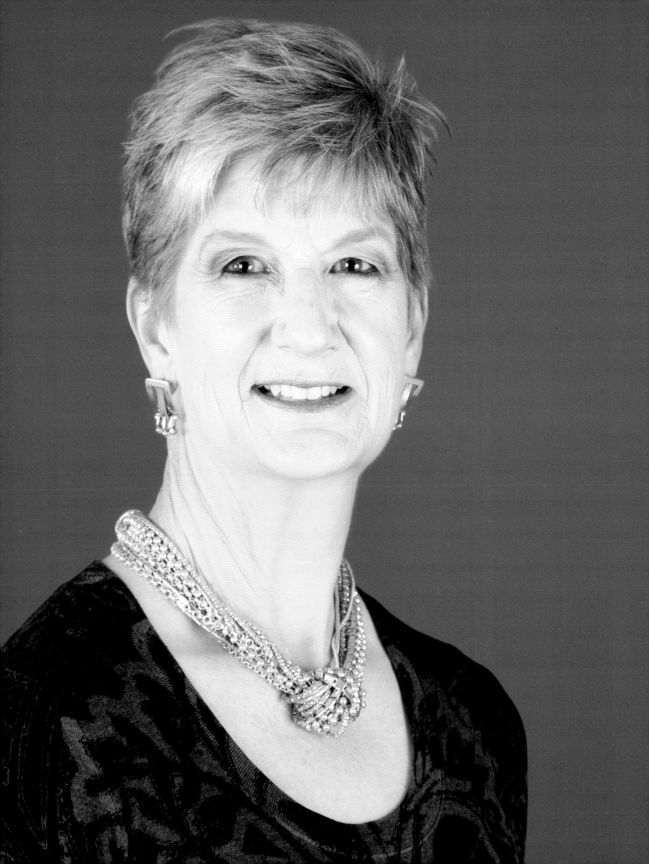

HALLIE

WRITER AND WORLD TRAVELER

Age: 72   Height: 5' 7"

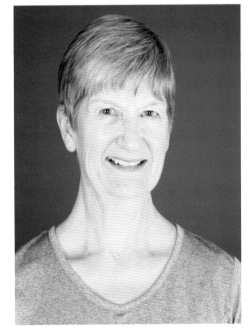

As a child Hallie spent most of her time in the fields and forests of the Pacific Northwest, where her Finnish father was an independent logger. She stayed on the West Coast throughout her time at university, earning her bachelor's and master's degrees, as well as membership in Phi Beta Kappa, at Stanford and Antioch universities. Hallie taught college and high school English for many years in the San Francisco Bay Area and internationally in Singapore, Brazil, and the UK.

Lately, she has devoted her days to writing poetry and finishing a spiritual memoir. Her poetry chapbook *So Many Gods* was the 2012 Blue Light Press contest winner. Hallie also received Rice University's Writer's Conference poetry prize in 1995; in 2013 she was awarded an art residency at Hilmsen Atelier in Salzwedel, Germany.

Hallie likes being active, waking early to meditate, walking a couple of miles with her dog, and spending time writing. She also takes Pilates classes to stay fit. Mother of three and a grandmother of four, she lives on her own with her dog, Sophie, north of Houston, Texas. Hallie is always open to new travel adventures and her desire to learn is insatiable. She recently found a way to combine her passions, using educational-travel nonprofit Road Scholar for its learning tours.

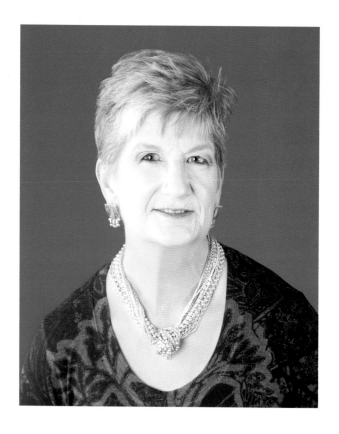

"Grace is a quality that comes almost unbidden. It is a blessing of sorts that if you maintain a demeanor and spirit receptive to grace, then **GRACE DESCENDS.**"

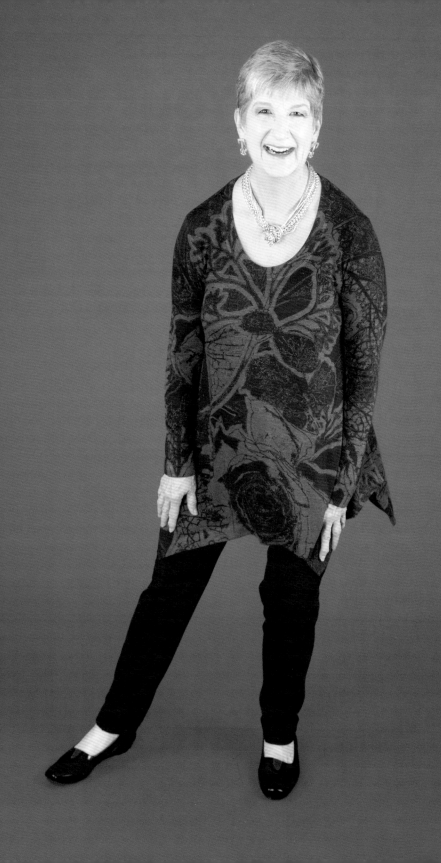

Eating Your Way to Good Health

KAREN RADEN, MS, RD, CCN

We are what we eat. Never is this old adage more important than as each birthday passes. Time puts heavy demands on the aging body. To stay healthy, we need to pay attention to how we are eating and supplement our bodies with proper nutrients.

Every passing year our bodies continue to break down. This may sound scary and depressing, but facing the truth allows us to use this knowledge to our advantage. In the aging process, free radicals accumulate and the inside of your body starts to, for lack of a better term, rust. Think of the "rusting" of our bodies as you would the engine of a car. Unless we care for our cars by providing proper fuel, routine checkups, and regular maintenance, rust will accumulate. Our bodies require similar care. While free radicals are not all bad, a buildup of too many in the body has been linked to specific diseases. If we do nothing to slow this progression, we are likely to age more quickly than is necessary.

Luckily, modern science teaches us that if we focus on our health, we can slow down the aging process. To this end, several key pieces of health advice apply to every mature woman:

> Modern science teaches us that if we focus on our health, **WE CAN SLOW DOWN THE AGING PROCESS.**

- Reduce inflammation.

- Maintain an ideal body weight.

- Support bone health.

- Support proper digestion.

I continually recommend these four essential guidelines, and my patients find themselves looking and feeling younger even as the years pass.

Reduce Inflammation

The topic of inflammation has recently become one of science's primary concerns. Inflammation falls into two basic types: acute and chronic. *Acute inflammation* happens when there is an immediate injury or wound that must be healed. When you cut yourself, for example, white blood cells and other "fighter cells" go to the area of the body in need of healing and try to mend it. The body works hard, employing various complicated and beautifully intricate biochemical reactions. This function is crucial for proper healing.

Chronic inflammation is a different story. Termed by many experts as a "slow-burning fire," it can continue in the body for many years on end. No injury has actually occurred, but the body thinks one has, so it produces an ongoing signaling mechanism that continues to fight off potential invaders. The "fire" never gets put out completely, but the immune system continues to try. Side effects of this ongoing assault can cause issues with various parts of your body:

- Your intestinal tract, leading to digestive issues

- Your joints, leading to arthritis and joint pain

- Your blood vessels, leading to atherosclerosis

Other consequences of inflammation may include certain cancers, diabetes, fibromyalgia, and Alzheimer's.

Unfortunately, many people do not even know they have chronic inflammation. Your physician can administer a C-reactive protein (CRP) test to determine whether your body suffers from chronic inflammation.

Given the stressful and toxic lifestyle common to the modern age, it is never too late to start trying to reduce inflammation.

There are several ways you can help your body do this.

EAT MORE FRESH FRUITS AND VEGETABLES

Research has shown that the antioxidants and phytonutrients (plant nutrients) present in fresh fruits and vegetables can help reduce inflammation in the human body. Try to incorporate some fresh, basic foods into your daily diet—frozen fruits and vegetables work too. Start by shopping for whole foods, making sure that the only ingredient in each item you are buying is the actual ingredient you want to eat. Avoid prepared and processed items that have unnecessary additives such as salt, sugar, fillers, and artificial colorings. A goal of six to nine servings of fruits and/or vegetables a day is ideal!

GET THE RIGHT FATS IN YOUR DIET

There are many misconceptions about acceptable fats in your diet. In fact, the type of fat you are ingesting is as important as the amount. It is crucial for the healthy body to get some fat daily. The right types of fat not only lubricate the body but also reduce inflammation. Women who do not eat enough fat may have dry skin, quicker wrinkling, and constipation.

The key is to focus on healthy fats such as those found in nuts, seeds, avocados, and olive oil. These are chiefly monounsaturated fats, which are good for your heart, your skin, and your whole body. Plus, make sure to get some omega-3 fatty acids daily. Found in wild-caught salmon, walnuts, flaxseed, and organic flax oil, omega-3s are essential to any effort to reduce inflammation in the body. Also important is the elimination from your diet of all trans fats, which are made synthetically from partially hydrogenated fats and are used in processed foods and commercial fried foods.

REDUCE SUGAR AND REFINED CARBOHYDRATES

Research has shown that too much sugar can also cause inflammation. Avoid foods with more than 10 grams of sugar per serving. Center your diet around whole foods: fruits, vegetables, nuts, seeds, whole grains, lean animal protein, and calcium-rich foods. **Avoid foods that contain high-fructose corn syrup, which promotes inflammation.**

INCORPORATE DIETARY SUPPLEMENTS

It is always important to consult a knowledgeable health-care professional before starting to take supplements. Some of my favorites that reduce inflammation are turmeric, fish oils, Boswellia, and mixed tocopherols. A nutritionist can suggest healthy amounts and forms for your needs.

Maintain an Ideal Body Weight

While many of us want to stay lean for reasons of vanity, the truth is that too much body fat can be inflammatory and cause premature aging. For most people, the higher our body fat percentage, the less healthy our body is. Although most of us do not have access to body fat testing, one simple way to determine if you are carrying too much fat is to use a simple calculation called the body mass index (BMI). There are many websites that will calculate this for you simply by using your height and weight.

If your BMI is not within the normal range, you may want to focus on strategies to reduce your weight and body fat.

Here are three weight loss tips that work:

1. **Never eat carbohydrates alone.** Pair your carbohydrates each time with protein and/or a healthy fat. This will help balance your blood sugar so you are not as hungry. Simple pairings could be rice cakes with peanut butter or an apple with cheese.

2. **Eat every three or four hours to prevent hunger.** The easiest way to gain weight is to get very hungry and then overeat.

3. **Stop eating two hours before you go to bed.** This allows your body time to heal while you sleep and forces it to use fat stores for fuel.

Support Bone Health

Women age sixty and over should consume 1,200 milligrams of calcium per day. Eating calcium-rich foods such as yogurt, cheese, cow's milk, and nondairy sources (hemp milk, broccoli, tahini, etc.) can add a great deal of calcium to your diet.

If you choose to supplement calcium, include at least some magnesium and vitamin D. Many women find that calcium supplements cause constipation; magnesium can offset this. I recommend that my patients have their vitamin D levels tested at least twice a year to determine the appropriate dosage for them to take.

Support Proper Digestion

Issues with digestion can pop up at any time of life. As we age, we tend to notice more physical ailments than when we were younger. The body tolerates less "abuse" as the years go on and it becomes worn out and tired. Moderating intake of late-night pizza and supersized coffee is a must for my patients who want to maintain their youthful healthy glow and keep their digestion functioning properly.

To promote healthy digestion with daily elimination, heed and follow these recommendations:

1. **Make sure to get enough water and fiber.** Many people start increasing their fiber intake to help with regularity; however, they forget to increase their water consumption as well. If you increase your fiber without increasing your fluid intake, you are creating a sponge in your body that can actually lead to more constipation. A good rule is to eat 25 grams of fiber per day and drink half your body weight in ounces of fluids.

> The body tolerates less "abuse" as the years go on and it becomes **WORN OUT AND TIRED.**

2. **Sip on hot lemon water with a little stevia or honey in the morning.** This great trick will help get peristalsis (i.e., speeding up the bowels) started and get the digestive tract moving, promoting easier elimination of waste from the body.

3. **Take a probiotic supplement.** Probiotics feed the good bacteria in your system. Many people who have digestive issues lack enough good bacteria in their body. This deficiency might stem from excessive antibiotic use, poor diet, and/or not enough fiber. Probiotics found in capsule form or in good-quality yogurt or kefir drinks can support the immune system. Probiotics can also alleviate suffering from a number of digestive ailments, including gas, bloating, diarrhea, and constipation.

Thoughtful food choices make a healthy and attractive body possible at any age. Inform yourself about nutrition—it's an important part of healthy aging.

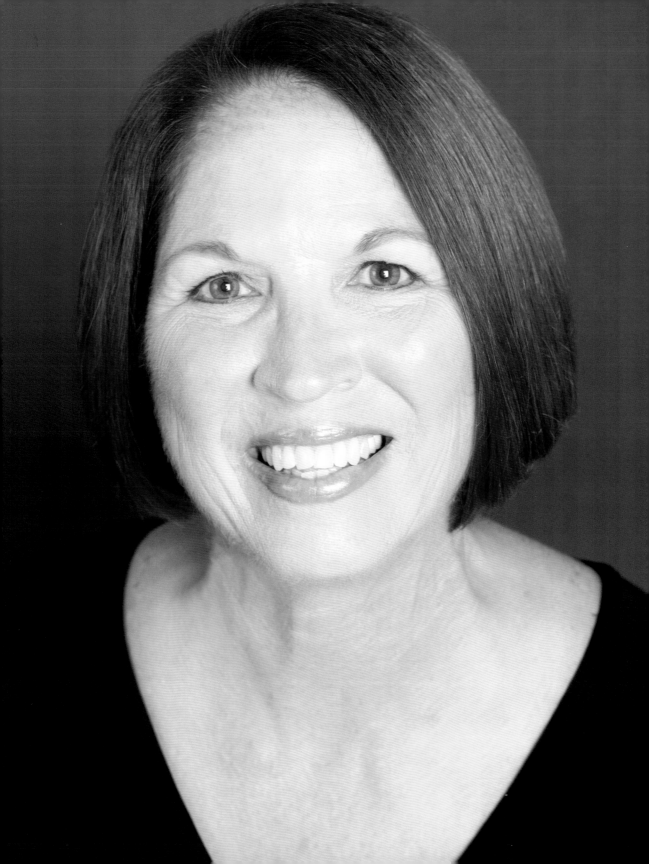

MARY JANE

EDUCATOR AND TIRELESS ORGANIZER

Age: 64   Height: 5' 6"

Mary Jane was born into a large Catholic family in New Orleans. She and her five siblings were raised in a three-bedroom, one-bath house that was under water after Hurricane Katrina hit the Crescent City. Mary Jane received her bachelor's in education and a master's in supervision administration. She taught social studies, physical education, and driver's education in Louisiana until 1981, when she moved to Denver with her new husband. There she served as an assistant principal at a local school.

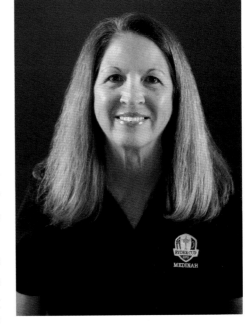

Caring for aging parents is a job no one is trained for, but Mary Jane moved to Texas in 1998 to do just that. She realized that her parents had given so generously and unconditionally of their love, time, and talents, and she was happy to give back to them. Mary Jane selflessly dedicated three years of her life to this loving task.

Once she retired from teaching, she began volunteering to assist with golf events. She has coordinated hundreds of volunteer workers for the PGA, AJGA, and the Champions Tour tournaments; her talents in supervision administration make her an essential member of the professional golf community. Mary Jane also loves to play golf, cook, listen to bluegrass music, and meet new people.

Mary Jane does not have children of her own, but feels lucky to figure in the happy memories of many former students scattered around the country. Through the Internet, students have reconnected with her and remain in touch.

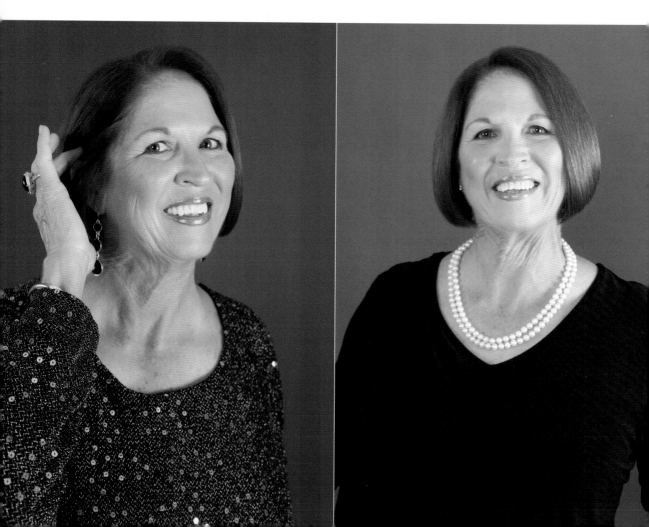

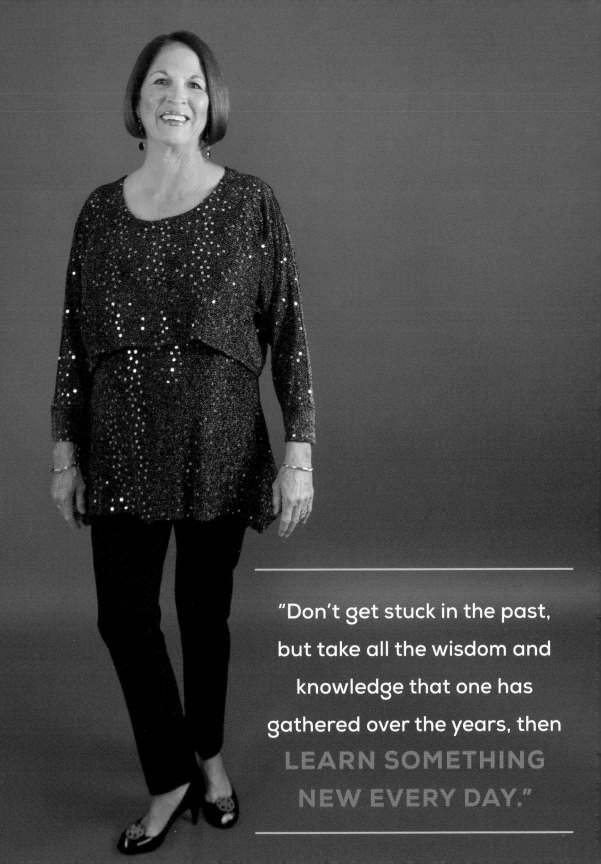

"Don't get stuck in the past, but take all the wisdom and knowledge that one has gathered over the years, then LEARN SOMETHING NEW EVERY DAY."

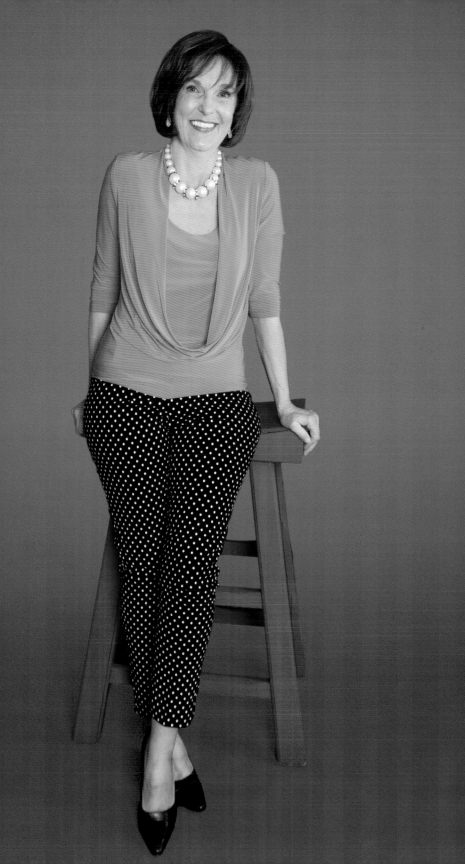

PAULA

ADVOCATE FOR AT-RISK YOUTH

Age: 71   Height: 5' 5"

Paula was born in Pittsburgh, where she and her brother and sister were lucky to be raised by two loving and devoted parents. The Steel City was Paula's home for twenty-seven years. At age seventeen, she entered the workplace as an executive secretary. That career path lasted six years, coming to an end with the arrival of twin boys. Shortly after, she and her husband also welcomed two new daughters. Paula's husband's work took the family to Denver, Texas, California, and Alberta, Canada.

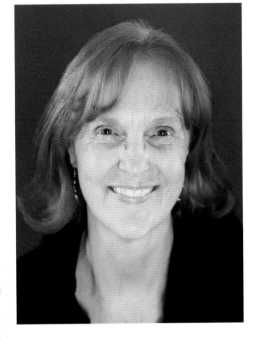

Paula's daughters both settled near their parents and have given her the pleasure of having three delightful grandsons. Paula's twin boys now live in Japan and she laments that she sees them infrequently. As an empty nester, Paula felt the desire to be more engaged and decided to put her energies into a volunteer program. She worked to improve quality of life for people with special needs through therapeutic horsemanship activities and education. She had no equestrian experience and the endeavor was a stretch for a city gal, but she was drawn to the challenge. Paula worked primarily with

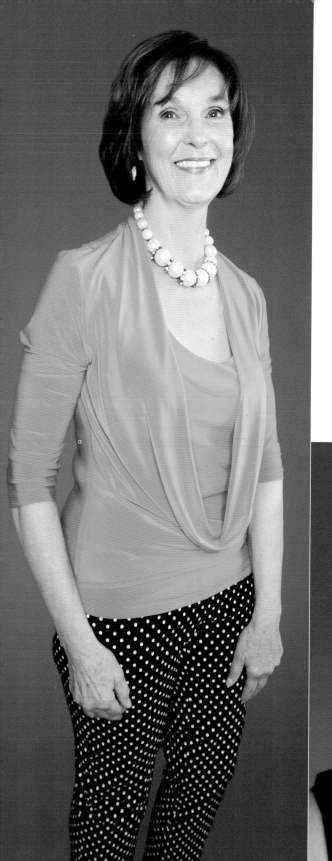

young children, staying beside the horse and securing the rider. Through the years, she felt privileged to see the children's progress and, at times, miracles.

She now mentors at-risk children in a school environment. This presents a different set of obstacles from those in her previous, more physical volunteer work. The mission here is to build a caring relationship and commit to working with one child on a weekly basis, helping with emotional, social, and academic needs. Paula is now in her third year with her mentee. She also stays physically active by participating in senior Pilates at the YMCA and traveling with her husband.

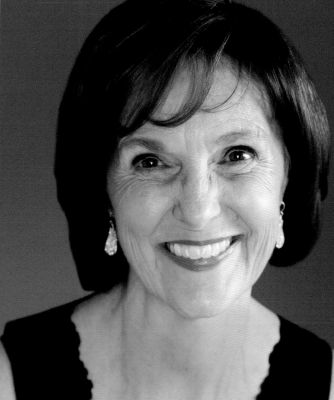

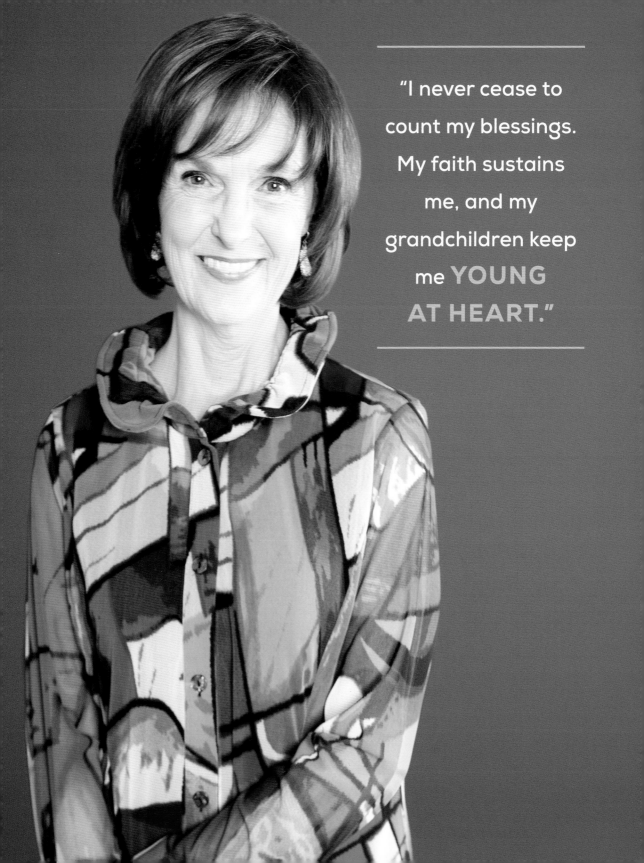

"I never cease to count my blessings. My faith sustains me, and my grandchildren keep me **YOUNG AT HEART.**"

How to Find the Strength to Regain Your Strength

**SANDRA SUTHERLAND,
CERTIFIED PERSONAL TRAINER**

When it comes to taking care of ourselves—body, mind, and spirit—we know what we are supposed to do in the fitness department. We are told to make time for cardio activity, strength training with weights, and flexibility exercises for overall balance. We might even have all the necessary tools to do those things. But at the end of the day, we find ourselves back where we started: seeking basic exercises that will give us strength daily.

Strength is what happens while you're doing something else, something so common that you probably didn't even notice you were building muscle tone and stamina. In fact, you can create new habits and convert task repetition into physical exercise even as your normal day goes on. Start by adding small movements to your daily routine to accomplish the BASICS: Balance, Abdominals, Strength, Intervals, Cardio, and Stretches.

The BASICS can all be done at home on a regular basis, just like your other everyday tasks: getting out of bed, getting dressed, brushing your teeth, brushing your hair . . . Simply add these exercises until they become a normal part of your day.

START BY ADDING SMALL MOVEMENTS to your daily routine to accomplish the BASICS: Balance, Abdominals, Strength, Intervals, Cardio, and Stretches.

Begin with bed *stretches*. Before you even take the first step out of bed, stretch your body completely, from head to toe. Reach upward toward the ceiling with your arms, and elongate your legs. Stretch as much as you need to in order to get the blood flowing, each day adding more time as required to take those first steps in the right direction. Then, as you slowly, deliberately sit up in bed, be conscious of how you feel within your skin. **Create an awareness of the whole body. Take inventory!**

As you rolled up to a sitting position, you used your *abdominal* muscles. You can repeat this movement for abdominal strength. Plus, your abdominals engage your back's muscles, and when these two systems work together, the entire core is present and getting stronger.

Take a deep breath now and *balance* yourself as you come out of bed. In a standing position reach up and stretch your arms toward the ceiling, then to your sides. Lean side to side with outstretched arms. Then, if possible, squat deeply, bending at your knees, to a sitting position. Hold this position for balance, then gradually bring yourself up to standing. Use squats to strengthen your core throughout the day and to protect the back in any lifting movements. You will use many muscles in the squat, so move slowly up and down to strengthen your quads, glutes, and core. As you become comfortable with the movements you will feel your muscles help in every stage.

Strength **is happening all day long.** Some examples include squatting in the kitchen to reach an item under the sink and lifting towels to put them away in the linen closet. You might never have noticed it before, but these movements are building strength! If you repeat the squatting motion eight to ten times, you are strengthening the legs; the lifting motion strengthens the arms. Even walking up the stairs in your home or when you are out and about can strengthen your quads, which help your knees do their job. Just remember to lift your feet with care to assure clearance, and repeat with confidence.

Deciding how to *think* during exercise is the most important part. While lifting that luggage or grabbing those grocery bags, it's easy to use only the bicep or shoulder rotator cuff. **Remind yourself to take notice of how your entire body is working to create movement and to protect your muscles from any jerking movements.** Think of the machinery within the body that goes into each movement. Using your core to aid the lift encourages full-body strength.

As you add little bits of motion here and there to your daily routine, it is essential to include a workout for the heart too. Do some cardio exercise to keep it ticking strong! Let your breathing be your guide. When it becomes difficult to speak, you have

> Think of the **MACHINERY WITHIN THE BODY** that goes into each movement. Using your core to aid the lift encourages full-body strength.

reached the hard level. Slow down, allowing your breathing to recover until you have reached easy. If you're out for a walk, speed up for a minute and then walk easy for the next two. Or set a goal— walk quickly until you reach the next traffic light or lamppost, and then move more slowly with easy effort until the next one. **An aerobic exercise time of twenty to forty minutes, three to five times a week will keep you feeling good and young for many years to come.** You pick: walking, running, cycling, swimming, dancing— they are all good.

Deciding **HOW TO THINK** during exercise is the most important part.

Work out in *intervals* to allow your heart to recover. Once your heart rate and breathing are back to normal, repeat the action. This can happen on a bicycle, in a pool, at the gym, on a home treadmill, or really with any type of exercise. Think, "One minute fast, two to three slow and easy." Give yourself more time to recover at first, and gradually increase the speedy periods as you reduce recovery time.

Finally, return to *stretching*—the feel-good exercise that is so important for the joints and muscles to keep them long and lean and easy to use. Apply your BASICS daily and see and feel the difference! Special tools can aid your progress. Those might include a pedometer, a small medicine ball, or a partner to exercise with—or join a group. Get out, breathe the fresh air, and get your day going! A daily walk, housecleaning, gardening, and other small tasks will use your muscles and increase strength as you use them. Remember to think about what muscles you will engage, use your core with any lifts, and move slowly to prevent injury. The best way to stay strong is to choose to move. Now go out and regain your strength!

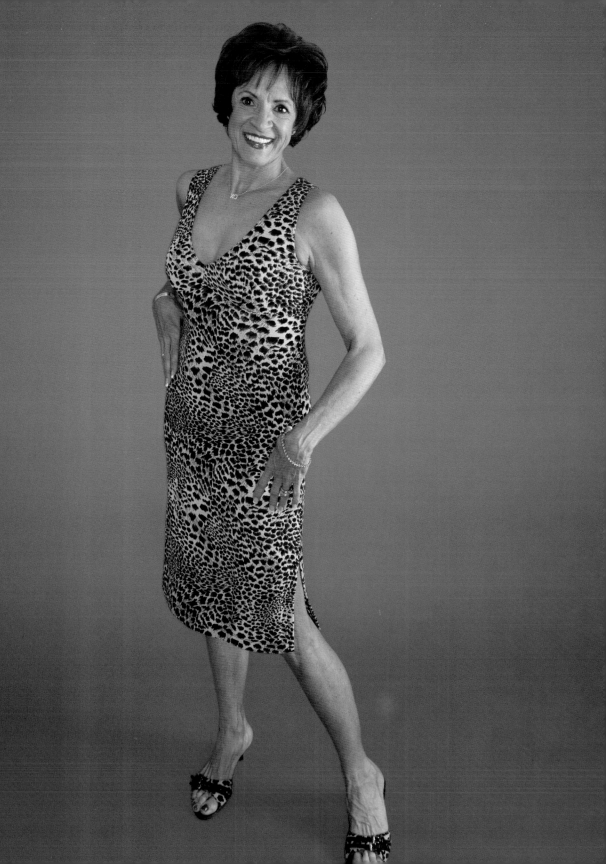

LYLETTE

UNSTOPPABLE FORCE AND ENTREPRENEUR

Age: 64   Height: 5' 7"

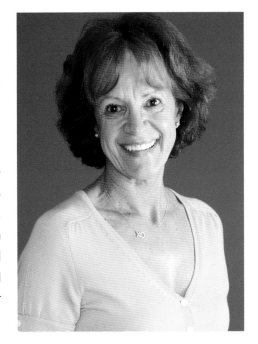

Lylette grew up on a midwestern military academy campus, where she learned etiquette, ballroom dancing, diving, horseback riding, and skeet shooting. She was the first female to attend the academy. The day after her high school graduation, she moved to New York to become a TWA stewardess. After furlough from TWA, she returned to the Midwest, married, and relished her life as an extremely involved stay-at-home mother. Years later, her husband was convicted of a white-collar crime. Lylette wished she had better work experience so that she could be more prepared to provide for her four children.

Her cars and home were repossessed. Although she had only "flight attendant" on her resume, Lylette found a position as a pharmacy technician and, eventually, pharmacy manager. She then moved into the construction contracting business, starting

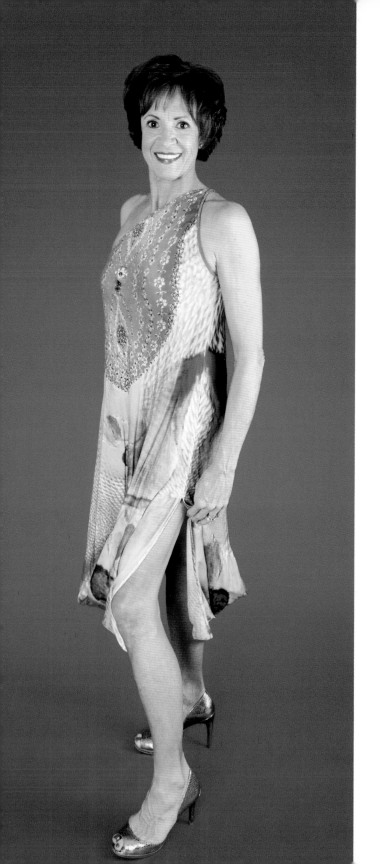

out as an assistant at a company and finally owning her own contracting company. Her tenacity is evident in her accomplishments, and she credits much of her success to those who helped her and her children when things were at their worst. During those hard times, she reminded her kids to "hold on to your family, your faith, and your education, because no one can take those things from you."

Though she divorced her husband immediately following his conviction, she remained dear friends with him until his death twenty years later. It was important for her to maintain a relationship for their children's sake. Lylette remarried recently, rekindling the flame with her high school crush, who asked her to attend their class reunion with him. Between the two of them, they have seven children and nine grandchildren. For his work they relocated to Texas, where Lylette established and leads a woman-owned small business dealing in atmospheric water generators, fuel cells, and modular buildings.

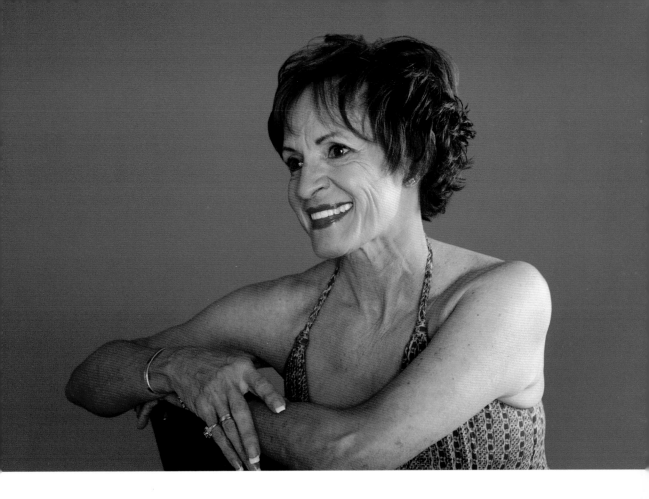

"**HOLD ON TO YOUR FAMILY,** your faith, and your education, because no one can take those things from you."

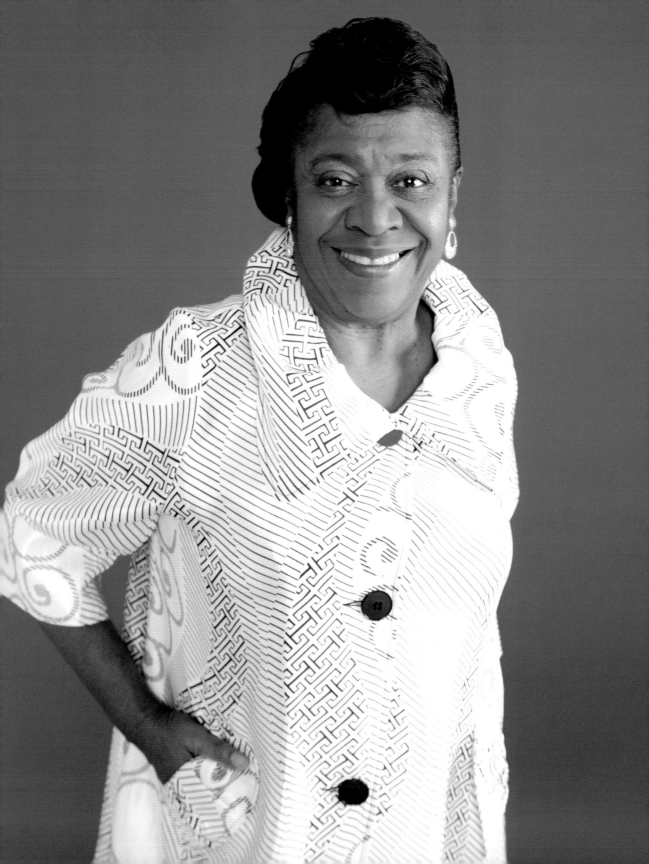

SAMMIE

ARDENT EDUCATOR AND HUMBLE SOUL

Age: 70   Height: 5' 6"

Sammie's parents taught her that God, family, and her fellow humans should be viewed with the utmost respect. They revered those who seek knowledge, and they often reminded Sammie that she should not only strive to do well for herself but also serve others. These values affected Sammie greatly and influenced her decision to be a teacher.

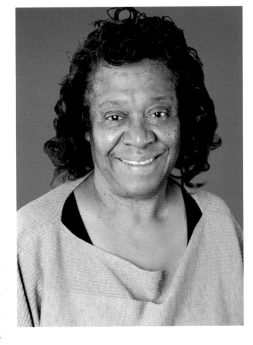

Once she graduated from college and began teaching, she was happy to find that she was living her passion daily. She took great pleasure in helping children realize their success. Sammie's greatest honor was being named Teacher of the Year at the elementary school where she taught. She has led a blessed life, was married, and had a wonderful family. When her middle child was diagnosed with a severe mental health problem, Sammie felt her courage dwindling. She didn't feel prepared to deal with the devastating disease that had suddenly entered her family's life. With some soul-searching and a lot of support from friends, family, her church, and her school family, she was able to find strength when faced

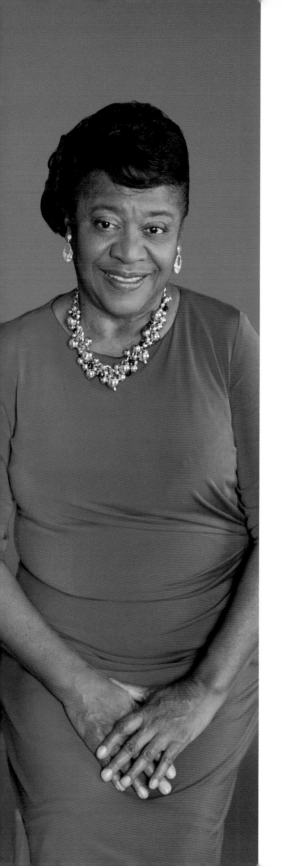

with the pain and confusion of watching her child suffer. When her husband died suddenly, she again had a strong community of caring people to help her through. She was grateful to have her children and students to lift her spirit.

Sammie taught for many years and learned that the key to being a successful teacher was to connect with and nurture each child as if that child were her own. Her heart was big enough to receive every student, and she let all of them know they were important and loved. In turn, each child was willing to do the best job that he or she could do. She is now retired from teaching, but she spends much of her time volunteering and working to help her three grandchildren be the best that they can be.

"As for me, **I WON'T SIT DOWN.** I will keep working and trying to help others to see the best in themselves. I will keep the vision that my parents instilled in me. I will **continue to love and respect God, my family, and my fellow man.**"

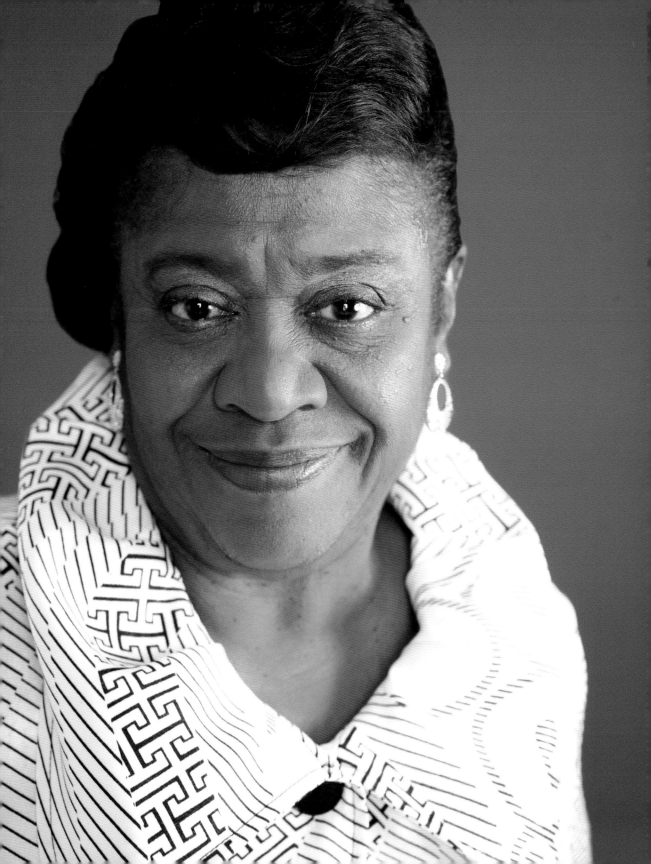

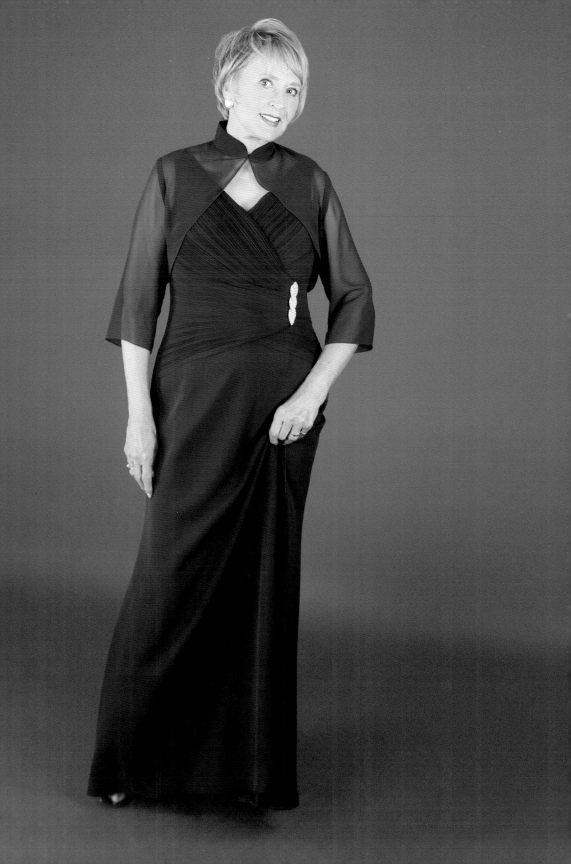

STAR

ACCOMPLISHED BUSINESSWOMAN AND ADVENTUROUS TRAVELER

Age: 71   Height: 5' 8"

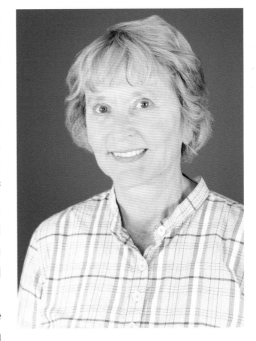

Star is a remarkably well-traveled woman who spent twenty years in Asia with her husband and two sons. While abroad she and her family happily welcomed the addition of two adopted daughters.

In Hong Kong, Star and a group of fellow teachers from the international school took a class in pearl knotting, which sparked an enthusiasm for beading. She found herself collecting interesting beads and stones in her travels. When Star and her family moved back to the States, she used her teaching skills to lead beading classes in and around Washington, DC.

Noticing the lack of a bead store in the area, Star decided to fill that void, opening one in the basement of her home. She invited talented jewelry design-ers to teach classes there, and soon she had buyers seeking out qual-ity beads at her weekly open house. Ten years later, her business had

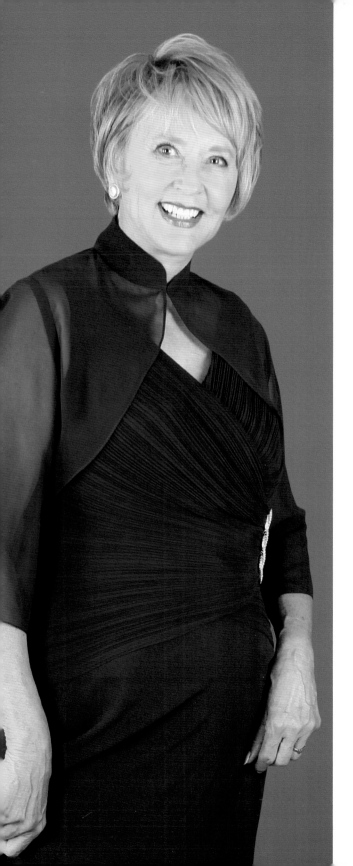

expanded beyond the capacity of her basement, and she opened a commercial space in Vienna, Virginia. Soon she was leading trips that introduced other bead enthusiasts to the wonders of markets and bazaars in Thailand, India, Morocco, Russia, Turkey, and Peru. In relatively little time, Star had managed to parlay an enjoyable and sustaining hobby into an extremely successful company. Now her youngest daughter is running the family business—but Star still checks in weekly to stay in touch with the many customers who have become lifelong friends.

Star took up marathoning at age forty while living in Asia. Although she no longer runs marathons, she manages to keep active at the gym and on the golf course. She still travels the world, is constantly pursuing new interests, and keeps her energy high by keeping fit.

Here, Star is wearing a flattering, elegant mother-of-the-bride gown, which she wore to her daughter's wedding.

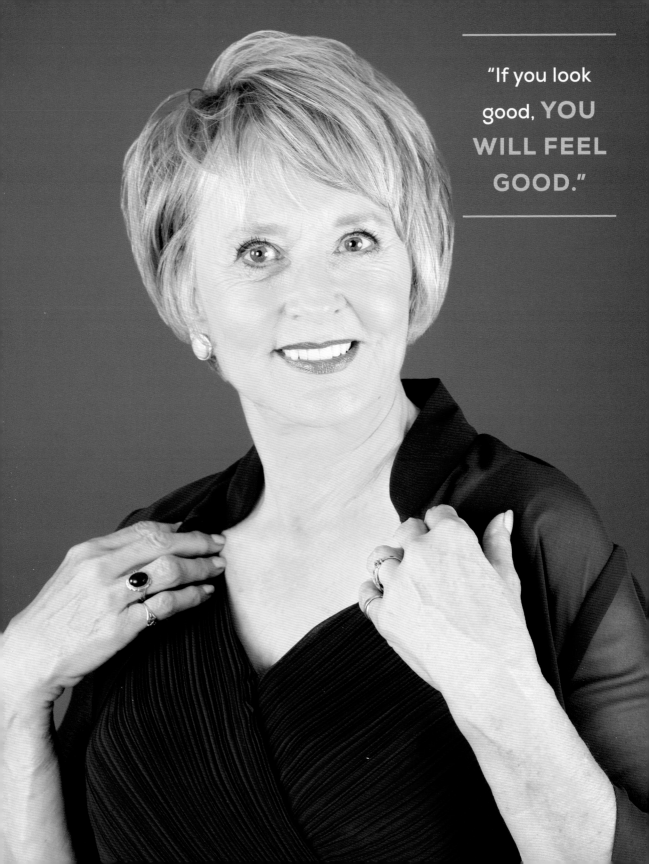

"If you look
good, **YOU
WILL FEEL
GOOD.**"

Looking Good

TOM H. SUN, MD

BOARD CERTIFIED OPHTHALMOLOGIST

As we find ourselves getting on in years, we must take steps to ensure that we continue "looking good"—not just in terms of appearance, but in a more literal, active sense. Good vision is essential to all our daily activities. **Poor vision compromises even the smallest pleasures of life, such as walking, eating, and sharing time with friends.** But serious vision problems for aging eyes are not a foregone conclusion. There are steps we can take now to prevent diseases that may worsen our vision.

Luckily, most choices that are good for the rest of the body are also good for the eyes. Good nutrition is vital. Exercise and a healthy weight protect good vision as well as overall health. Smoking may increase vision risks. Make an annual checkup with a vision professional. And by all means, wear sunglasses to protect your eyes against ultraviolet rays. Such eye protection reduces the likelihood of skin cancers on lids and also growths (pterygiums) on the actual eye surface itself. Just as significant, shielding the eyes with dark glasses has been shown to offer some benefit in preventing age-related macular degeneration and slowing cataract growth.

In many instances, current medical practice can provide effective treatment for the following debilitating maladies. These are "the big three" that can disturb our vision as we get older—the most common conditions that affect our aging eyes.

Cataracts

Cataracts manifest as blurred vision when the eye's lens becomes progressively cloudier. All humans get cataracts with age, but treatment isn't needed until blurry vision interferes with our daily activities. **To treat cataracts, an ophthalmologist replaces your cloudy natural lens with a clear artificial lens that will never get cloudy.** Advancement in cataract surgery techniques in the last forty years has simplified this operation, reducing it to a ten- or twenty-minute procedure that is safer than ever before.

Glaucoma

Glaucoma occurs when the optic nerve is damaged. This results in progressive loss of peripheral vision. In severe cases, even central vision can be lost. **The major risk factor here is pressure inside the eye, which can lead**

Make an annual checkup with a vision professional. And by all means, **WEAR SUNGLASSES** to protect your eyes against ultraviolet rays.

> Although there are **INHERENT RISKS** that come with age, failing vision is by no means inevitable.

to permanent damage if left untreated. To check for glaucoma, in addition to checking your eye pressure, your ophthalmologist might examine the appearance of the optic disc, the complete field of vision, the angle in the eye where the iris meets the cornea, and the thickness of the cornea.

Most of the time glaucoma is painless, and a person with glaucoma will not notice anything wrong with her vision until there is irreversible damage. For this reason, regular eye exams are vital for diagnosis of glaucoma.

Age-Related Macular Degeneration (AMD)

The leading cause of vision loss in an aging population is macular degeneration, which happens when the center of the retina, called the macula, deteriorates. AMD impacts central vision, making independent activities such as driving and reading especially difficult. Blank spots appear on the page or the road; in the most advanced cases, a person will not be able to make out the big E on the eye chart.

Millions of older adults worldwide have one of two types of AMD. The first, termed "dry" macular degeneration, develops from deposits and/or pigment changes in the macula. The second type, termed "wet" macular degeneration, occurs when fluid leaks into the macula. This type of AMD causes more rapid vision loss. But the good news is, now there are medications that can be injected into the eye to stabilize and even improve vision. A thorough eye checkup can determine if you have AMD.

Preventing the Big Three

Although there are inherent risks that come with age, failing vision is by no means inevitable. What can you do to boost your protection? The most consistent treatment is a lifestyle that includes a regular exercise routine and a wholesome diet rich in certain foods that help support eye health. **Foods high in omega-3s—nuts, seeds, cold-water fish such as salmon and sardines—also help keep vision clear.** Your eye doctor may recommend high-potency antioxidant supplements to help guard against macular degeneration in aging eyes—so be sure to make him or her an important member of your health team.

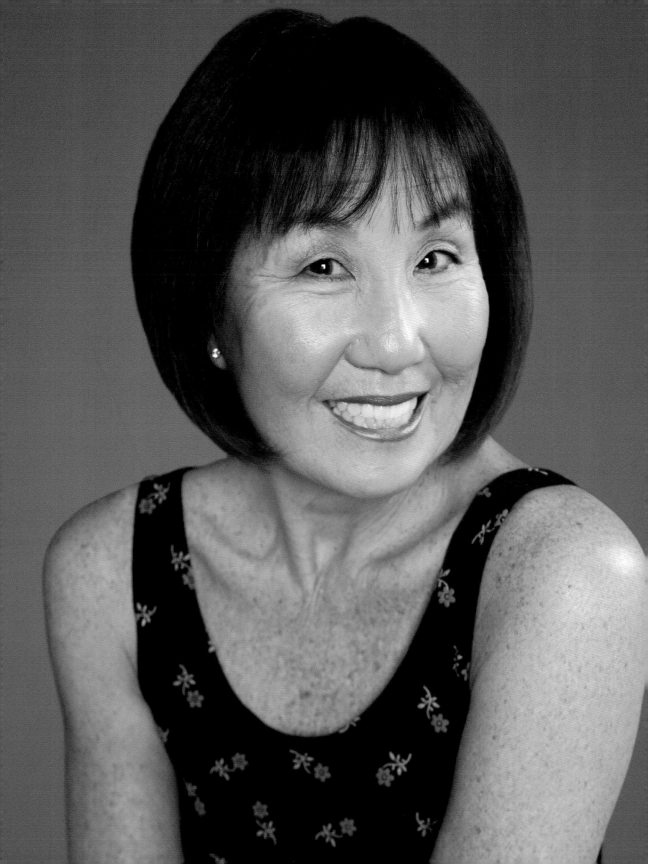

CAROL

FITNESS PIONEER AND INSPIRATIONAL LEADER

Age: 65   Height: 5' 3"

Carol joined a local swim team at age nine and has continued to compete in swim events for the last fifty-six years. She has been nationally ranked in both indoor and rough-water courses and has taught and coached swimming for forty years, inspiring both young and mature students to swim well and powerfully. She has completed forty marathons in forty years; in 1977 she was the winner of the Primo 50-kilometer run. Every year on her birthday she completes a "birthday triathlon" wherein she adjusts the minutes spent on each event to match her number of years spent on this earth. So for her sixty-fifth birthday she runs, bikes, and swims for sixty-five minutes each without stopping to rest.

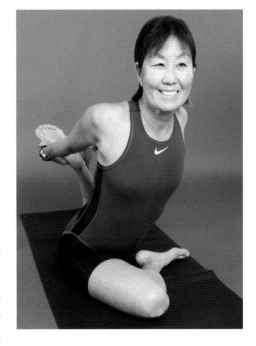

Carol received her bachelor's in education from the University of Hawaii and her master's in physical education and therapeutic recreation from Indiana State University. She has promoted wellness throughout

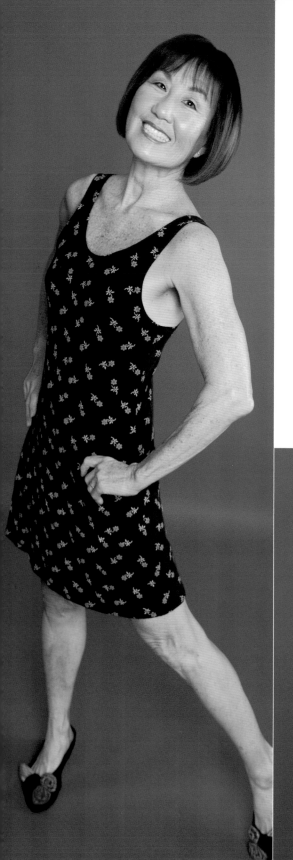

her years of working as an owner/operator of fitness centers in Southeast Asia. She motivated many members to lead a healthy life by incorporating good eating habits, exercise, and most of all a positive outlook into their everyday routine. Her fitness expertise opened the door for her to write health-related articles for magazines, appear as a frequent guest on radio talk shows, and host a fitness program on television.

Since retiring, she has helped empower female friends by leading weekly running sessions, aiding them in achieving their goals of finishing a full or half marathon. A few of her friends have even progressed to triathlon training. Carol feels blessed to be a survivor of ovarian cancer and firmly believes that "knowledge is power; attitude is everything."

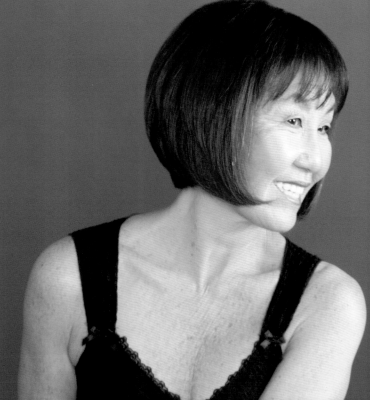

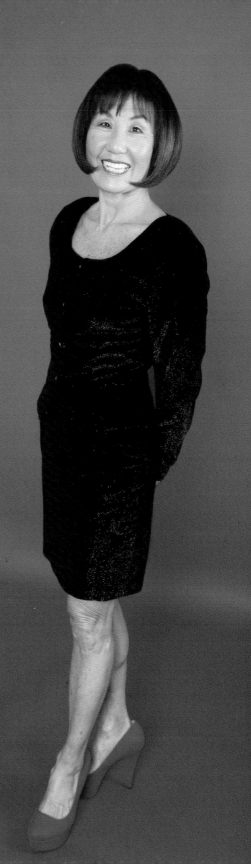

"ENGAGE IN PREVENTATIVE FITNESS rather than rehabilitative fitness."

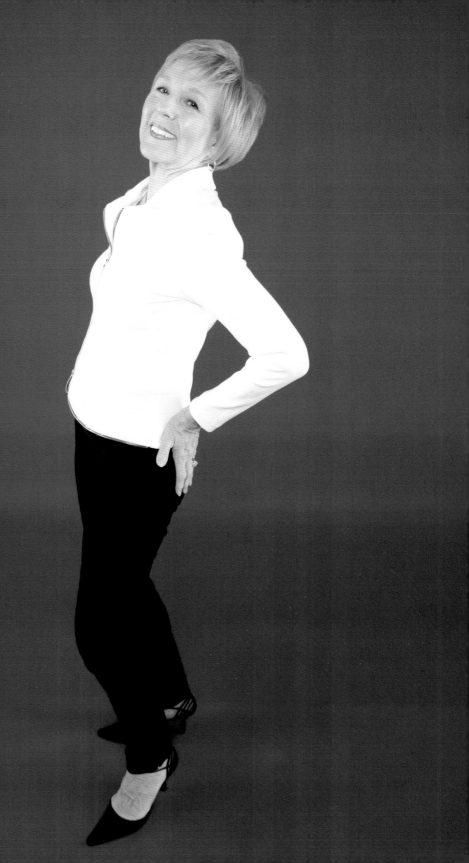

BARBARA

CAREER EXECUTIVE AND HOME RENOVATOR

Age: 71   Height: 5' 6"

Barbara was born the oldest of four children in St. Louis, Missouri. She met her husband of forty-seven years while they both worked for the same company. Early in her career, she had a supervisor who accepted nothing less than perfection, and that experience enriched Barbara's work ethic, causing her to do extensive research and double-check everything. While at a later point in her career, Barbara learned that appearance and attitude are just as important as skills and knowledge. Utilizing her newly acquired problem-solving and self-presentation skills, Barbara incorporated new techniques into her career and her personal life.

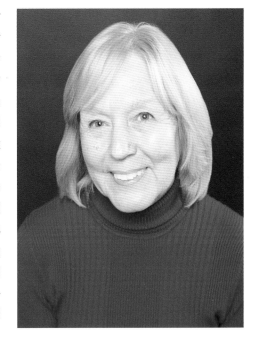

Four years later, the couple moved to Chicago and fell in love with the city. She began playing indoor tennis, as her preferred game of golf wasn't a possibility in Chicago's harsh winters. Barbara realized

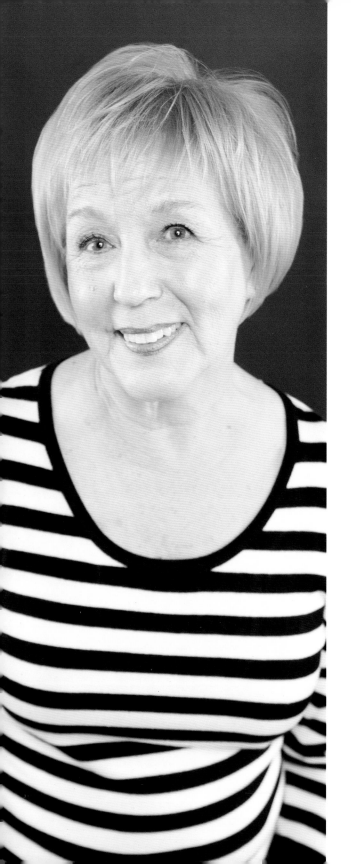

that playing sports was essential to living a healthy and socially active life. Next she found herself in Cleveland, where she met and became friends with a coworker's wife who was an interior designer. Barbara and her husband were living in a home built in the mid-1800s that was on the National Register of Historic Places. As they renovated the home, her new friend provided guidance. The couple taught themselves plumbing, electrical wiring, and all the necessary skills to do as much work as possible by themselves. To this day, she and her husband always keep an eye out for houses they can renovate and sell.

Barbara learned to appreciate the history and aesthetics of antiques and quality reproduction furniture. She renovated a piano that had been in the family since the early 1900s and decided to try something new—she learned how to play it.

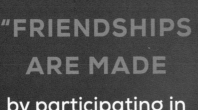

"**FRIENDSHIPS ARE MADE** by participating in activities and giving of yourself. Everyone wants friends; however, they will not come knocking on your door."

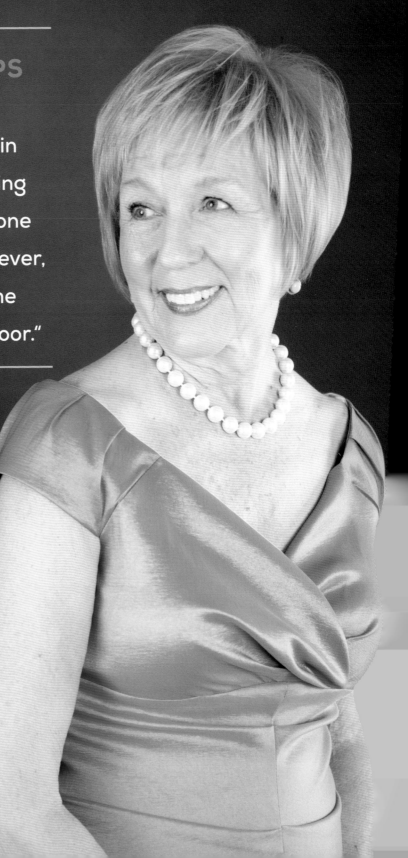

Modern Dentistry and Your Smile

WILLIAM C. WAMBAUGH, DDS

As we age, a bright smile with healthy teeth is one of the best accessories we have—a style we can continue to wear well. A recent survey noted that a person's smile is one of the first things we notice when meeting for the first time, regardless of age. The fact is, our teeth mature along with our bodies. Yet while tooth wear in older mouths is inevitable, a consistent daily hygiene routine, professional dental care, and possibly cosmetic and aesthetic improvement can ensure a confident smile.

Brush, Brush, Brush— Floss, Floss, Floss

Every daily routine should include the fundamentals of dental care: brushing and flossing. Most of us grew up with that directive as a key prescription for healthy teeth, but a reminder is always helpful.

Be conscientious about home dental care. Use a soft-bristle brush two or three times a day, and include your tongue in the brushing. The most important part of brushing our teeth is removing the bacteria from under the gumline and around our teeth. Most of us have a bit of gum tissue that is pliable and can readily harbor bacteria and food debris. The actual tooth itself is nearly self-cleaning.

Flossing—at least once a day—is also crucial to remove food debris. It can prevent tooth loss caused by gum problems such as gingivitis and periodontal disease, and it freshens your breath, too. Regular use of an oral irrigator (such as Waterpik) can also help keep gum tissue food-free and healthy. Many people avoid flossing or "forget" to floss, allowing bacteria to take hold and flourish. With prolonged neglect, bacteria will promote gum disease—the biggest cause of tooth loss after age fifty. The bacteria form plaque, which begin to erode the bone that stabilizes the tooth's roots. Eventually the gum

> A winning smile may be the height of fashion— but **BAD BREATH IS NEVER STYLISH.**

will deteriorate and even further bone erosion will occur.

Often a bleeding gum, discomfort at the gumline, or a sensitive tooth will alert us to a serious condition. Sometimes a tooth may even become loose. But even without this obvious sign, bone erosion may be happening: When plaque hardens into what is called "calculus," it can actually hold a tooth in place. **To address these problems, consider upgrading from a manual brush to an electric toothbrush.** It improves plaque removal, offers an easy way to massage the gums, and is easier to use for people with arthritis or other hand control issues.

A winning smile may be the height of fashion—but bad breath is never stylish. Besides food debris lingering between the teeth, another major cause of bad breath may be dry mouth provoked by medications that older people take to maintain their health. **I do not recommend strong mouthwashes, as they contain alcohol and other ingredients that tend to dry out the mouth and increase breath problems.** Frequent sips of water throughout the day help reduce dry mouth and freshen sour breath.

Excellent home care becomes critical in your efforts to prevent these issues from causing root decay and tooth loss. But don't forget to also stay current with dental visits. Regular dental checkups are vital even if you are not noticing a specific problem; if there is any bleeding or pain in the gums, a visit to the dentist is a must. Your teeth and gums need regular attention (a cleaning every six months) and regular X-rays (annually). **There is no substitute for the keen eye of your dental hygienist and dentist, who will evaluate your teeth and gums for signs of disease or decay, for any evidence of cancer of the tongue or mouth, and for overall oral health.** Our teeth may shift as we age, which affects bite and creates more wear on tooth surfaces. Dental professionals can evaluate your bite and keep it efficient. Make brushing and flossing part of your daily routine, and make time in your calendar for trips to the dentist. Losing teeth is not a general part of aging, but if we neglect good care and professional guidance, it can be.

Correcting with Fillings

Modern dentistry offers a vast array of solutions to address the problems of aging and problematic teeth. The familiar silver fillings of the past—actually a mixture of silver, tin, and mercury—today are replaced by tooth-colored fillings made of a composite of resins and glass ceramics that mimic your teeth. When bonded to the tooth, this filling forms a natural-looking restoration. As a bonus, these tooth-colored fillings can also be used to make lifelike replacements and cosmetic changes to the shape of the front teeth.

If your teeth are suffering from larger areas of decay or if a tooth has worn down so that your bite is affected, your dentist can create an onlay or a crown of either gold or ceramic. An onlay is bonded directly to the remaining tooth, while a crown covers the entire tooth above the gumline. The newer ceramic materials are strong and very lifelike, and they eliminate the dark lines seen at the gumline on older crowns. As with our own teeth, tooth-colored fillings can discolor due to food and drink staining. Coffee, tea, red wine, and tobacco are the chief culprits. Regular brushing and flossing helps keep fillings a shade of white that blends with your teeth.

Dealing with Tooth Loss

When teeth are lost due to decay, fracture, or gum disease, replacements are needed to fill the space for proper function and looks. There are several options: a bridge, an implant, or a partial denture. The specific tooth loss often dictates the choice of treatment. All result in a natural-looking replacement for the lost teeth.

A bridge is a fixed covering, like a crown, with a replacement "tooth" (or "teeth") connected between the two retaining teeth on either side. An implant replaces a single tooth with a titanium root, placed in the bone of the missing tooth space, and a crown placed on this root. A partial denture is a removable appliance held in place by clasps to the surrounding teeth. Each choice varies in flexibility, cost, and time needed to complete the treatment.

The process of aging is inevitable— **ALL TEETH WEAR DOWN.**

Adding Cosmetic Flourishes

In the last couple of decades tooth whitening, veneers, and orthodontia for adults have become common dental services. Over time our teeth can yellow, chip, and even crack, leaving us unsatisfied with our smile even when our teeth continue to function properly. Today's technological advances mean we can feel good about our smile again.

Whitening offers a noninvasive way to change tooth color without harming the tooth itself. The outpatient whitening process requires custom-made trays that cover the teeth and hold the whitening solution next to the teeth to remove stains. To gain maximum whitening, patients must have the trays in place five to six hours a day (typically during sleep) for two weeks. Dentists treat darker stains in the office using federally and professionally controlled solutions that require careful protection of the gums. Either way, this procedure produces dramatic results. On the other hand, most over-the-counter whitening products yield minimal results and probably are not a wise way to spend your time and money.

> It is not unusual these days to see an older adult in **BRACES.**

Veneers, made of porcelain, ceramic, or composite resin materials, have been around since the mid-1980s. They require some minimal removal of or change to the tooth structure before being bonded. Porcelain and ceramic veneers both give the most lifelike results and don't change color over the years. **Veneers can help you achieve a lovely smile and can last twelve to fifteen years, depending on wear.**

If drastic tooth removal or a realignment is required, orthodontics (braces) is a better choice. It is not unusual these days to see an older adult in braces.

A Partnership for Life

The process of aging is inevitable—all teeth wear down. But just because it happens to all of us doesn't mean we have to resign ourselves to an inferior smile. Establishing a health partnership with your dentist is part of the solution. Modern dentistry delivers care gently and comfortably, using state-of-the-art equipment to give you a healthy mouth and an attractive smile. With the advances in dentistry today, it is possible for you not only to keep your teeth for a lifetime but also to keep them beautiful.

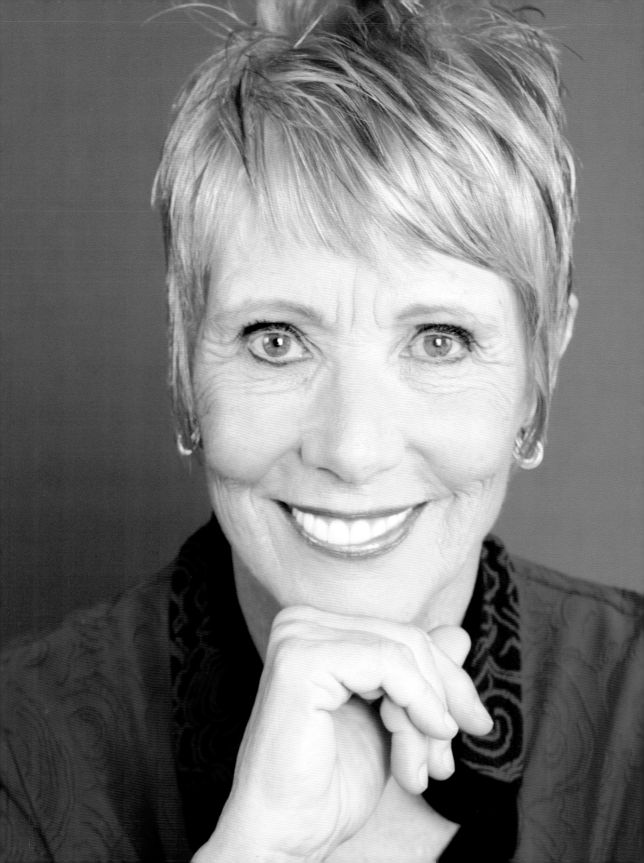

GERRIE

EQUESTRIAN ENTREPRENEUR

Age: 66   Height: 5' 8"

Gerrie's tenacity has served her well. She meets life with a positive attitude, and her enterprising nature has provided her with diverse life experience. Her career path is varied—she has owned not only a successful employment service but also a flourishing equestrian business.

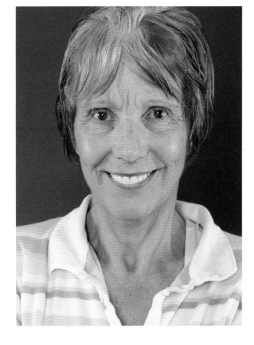

Gerrie recently studied for her real estate license, but after a few months in the real estate business she realized it might not be the best path for her. When she suddenly found herself in the midst of divorce after thirty-two years of marriage, she made a significant change: She picked up and moved from Colorado, leaving the real estate business, to Texas, where her son and his family live. There she moved into a home in a fifty-five-and-older community. Gerrie began searching for work in her new town but found it difficult, realizing that despite her qualifications, education, and experience, most employers do not typically hire older workers.

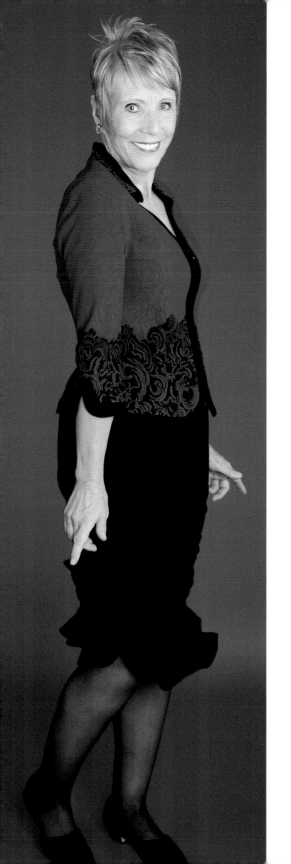

She remained optimistic and eventually decided to follow her dreams and resurrect the equestrian business she had enjoyed so much in the past.

She now happily spends her days giving riding lessons and training horses—her true passion. Gerrie is thrilled to have the chance to become more acquainted with her two young granddaughters. She enjoys her new community's many social opportunities. These recent life changes have clearly been a positive experience, allowing her to live her life to the fullest and pursue her passions. She leads a very active life and would like a sensible, fresh look that will improve her business image and give her the confidence to thrive in her newly single life.

"I WANT TO LOOK MATURE, yet 'plugged in,' without that look that says 'I'm trying too hard' or wearing age-inappropriate clothing."

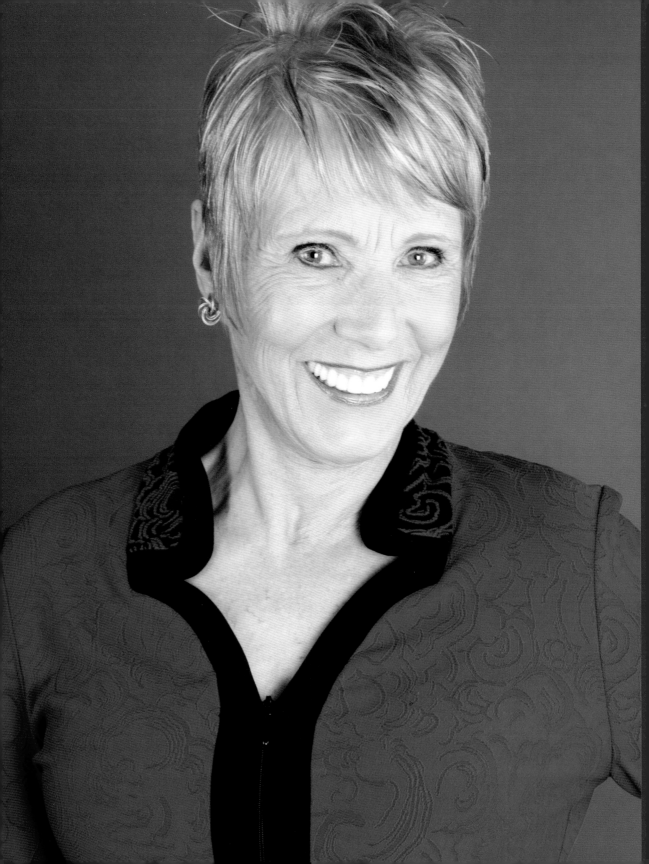

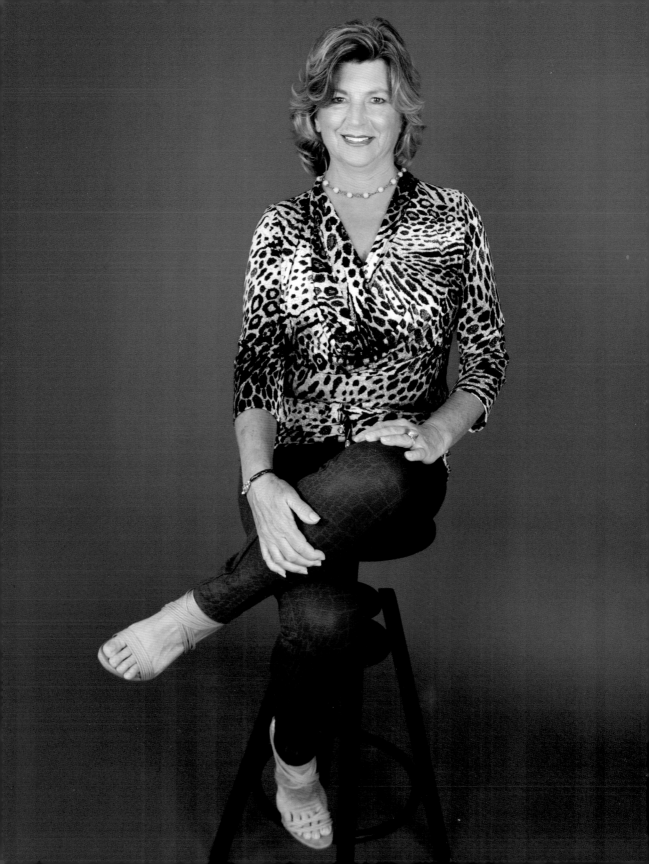

LYNN

FIRST WOMAN TO CAPTAIN A 747 ACROSS THE ATLANTIC

Age: 62   Height: 5' 4"

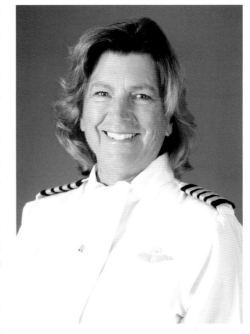

Lynn has spent the past thirty-six years as a commercial airline pilot. She and a colleague were the first women to captain a 747 across the Atlantic Ocean. Lynn began in aviation as a flight attendant and swiftly worked her way up, becoming the first flight attendant in history to earn a commercial pilot's license. Her accomplishments have been honored by the Smithsonian Institution, where her former uniform is on display. She appeared in the BBC documentary series *Reaching for the Skies* and was the first American to be designated Woman of the Year in England.

   As a single working mom, Lynn would fly during the week, scheduling her flights so that she would be home in time to share a family dinner with her sons. Now both her boys are off at college and Lynn is ready for a change. She is preparing to transition from her esteemed career in aviation to the world of corporate training, motivational speaking, and coaching.

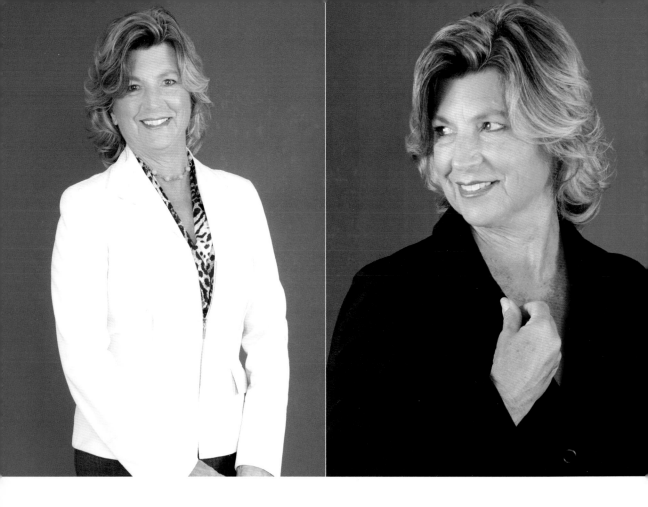

She will also be spending much of her time helping to establish a medical clinic on the island of Roatán, Honduras. Using her organizational skills from years in the cockpit, Lynn is solving some of the clinic's needs via the US-based organization Medical Bridges, which gives her access to surplus or donated medical equipment. Recently Lynn obtained an EKG machine—the first ever on the island. Her effort to upgrade the health of the Roatán population, in particular the poor, is a worthy goal for this skilled woman; her medical mission will change the lives of many residents. She is committed to finding funding, medical personnel, and volunteers to continue support for this humanitarian project.

Lynn has spent the majority of her life in a pilot's uniform and needs a new look for her stage presence as a public speaker, along with a comfortable warm-weather look and hairstyle for her work in Honduras.

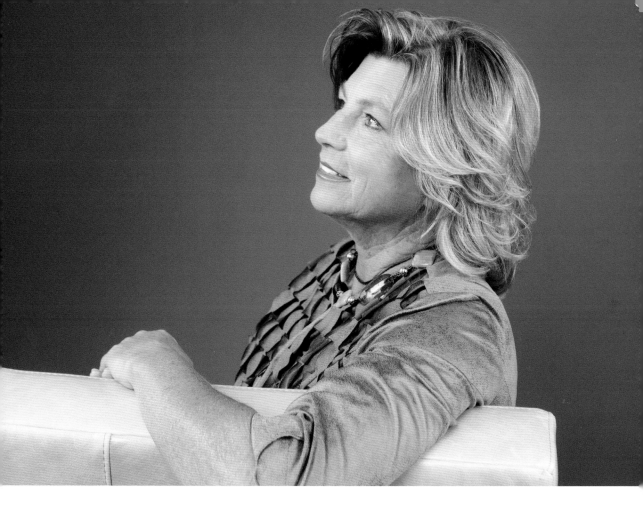

"Live without fear, be at peace with the past, and enjoy the present experience while **PLANNING THE NEXT ADVENTURE."**

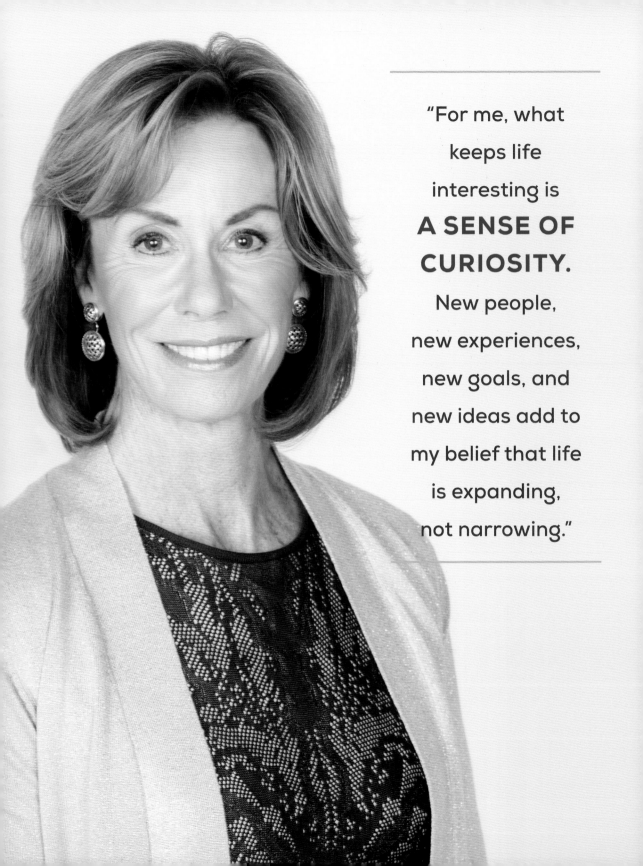

"For me, what keeps life interesting is **A SENSE OF CURIOSITY.** New people, new experiences, new goals, and new ideas add to my belief that life is expanding, not narrowing."

About the Author

ANNE REIZER, 70

During Anne Reizer's twenty-five years of living abroad in Asia and England, she has cultivated her unique style savvy through keen observation of timeless style and women who are active and confident in their maturity. Anne believes that polished personal style shines like a beacon and makes confident women distinctly visible.

Anne knows that exercise is vital to a positive attitude and believes in the importance of including physical fitness into her daily schedule. She counts a dozen treks to Nepal, many golf tournaments, and numerous marathons in her fitness dossier. She understands that with maturity comes the need to adjust fitness goals, but continues to pursue personal fitness and healthy living. Anne has enjoyed professional experiences as a teacher in the US and Asia and as a real estate agent.

Anne currently resides in Houston, Texas, and Breckenridge, Colorado.

About the Photographer

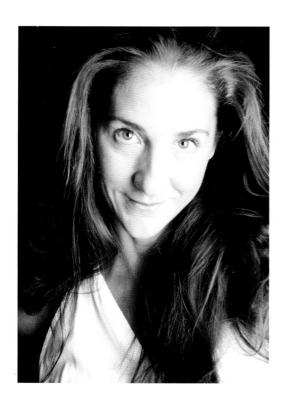

Gabriela Lavalle, a graduate of the National School of Bellas Artes in Mexico City, holds a photography degree from the National University of Belgium in Antwerp. A successful graphic reporter for lifestyle magazines and major newspapers in Mexico, Gabriela has directed the art photography of several marketing campaigns for national and multinational companies.

Acknowledgments

Anne Reizer would like to thank the following contributors to *Beautiful Encore*:

Karina Aureli

Wardrobe Stylist

Pamela Benison, MA

Fellow, American Psychotherapy
 Association
Denver, Colorado
pamelabenison.com

Joel Holland

Master Hairstylist
Sensia Studio & Spa
Houston, Texas
sensiastudio.com

Clint Johnson, MPT

Physical Therapist, Manager
Sterling Ridge Sports Medicine Center
The Woodlands, Texas
srosm.com

Magnena Jones

M Studio Hair Salon
The Woodlands, Texas
mstudiohairsalon.com

Sabrina A. Lahiri, MD, FACS.

Plastic and Reconstructive Surgery
Diplomate, American Board of Plastic
 Surgery
lahiriplasticsurgery.com

Gabriela Lavalle

Indivisible Art Projects

Patty Mansur

Wardrobe Stylist

Dr. Scott Marquardt, CCC-A, FAAA

Audiologist
The Woodlands, Texas
hearingwithclarity.com

Melissa McKinney

Makeup Artist
Sensia Studio & Spa
Houston, Texas
sensiastudio.com

Ivan Perez

Photo Editor

Karen Raden MS, RD, CCN

Integrated Nutritionist
Northbrook, Illinois
karenraden.com

Scruples Boutique

Houston, Texas
scrupleshouston.com

Stephen Strum

Owner, Sensia Studio & Spa
Houston, Texas
sensiastudio.com

Tom H. Sun, MD

Board Certified Ophthalmologist
Tomball, Texas
281-351-7483

Sandra Sutherland USAT, RRCA, PT

Fitness Consultant
Triathlon, Marathon, and Pilates Certified
The Woodlands, Texas
txtri.com

William C. Wambaugh, DDS

General and Cosmetic Dentistry
The Woodlands, Texas
dentistinthewoodlands.com